◆ 药学实验系列教材 ◆

药剂学
实验教程

Pharmaceutics Experiments Tutorial

胡海燕　吴传斌　主编

中山大学出版社
SUN YAT-SEN UNIVERSITY PRESS

·广州·

图书在版编目（CIP）数据

药剂学实验教程/胡海燕，吴传斌主编．—广州：中山大学出版社，2020.10
ISBN 978 - 7 - 306 - 06983 - 2

Ⅰ．①药…　Ⅱ．①胡…　②吴…　Ⅲ．①药剂学—实验—高等学校—教材
Ⅳ．①R94 - 33

中国版本图书馆 CIP 数据核字（2020）第 190406 号

YAOJIXUE SHIYAN JIAOCHENG

出 版 人：王天琪
策划编辑：陈　慧　谢贞静
责任编辑：谢贞静
封面设计：曾　婷
责任校对：梁嘉璐
责任技编：何雅涛
出版发行：中山大学出版社
电　　话：编辑部 020 - 84110771，84113349，84111997，84110779
　　　　　发行部 020 - 84111998，84111981，84111160
地　　址：广州市新港西路 135 号
邮　　编：510275　传　　真：020 - 84036565
网　　址：http：//www. zsup. com. cn　E-mail：zdcbs@ mail. sysu. edu. cn
印 刷 者：广州一龙印刷有限公司
规　　格：787mm × 1092mm　1/16　15 印张　400 千字
版次印次：2020 年 10 月第 1 版　2020 年 10 月第 1 次印刷
定　　价：40.00 元

本书编委会

主　编　胡海燕　吴传斌

编　委　（以姓氏拼音为序）

冯　敏　胡海燕　黄　莹　刘　丹

陆　超　潘　昕　权桂兰　吴传斌

徐月红　张雪飞　赵春顺

序

　　药剂学是研究药物制剂的基本理论、处方设计、制备工艺、质量控制和合理应用的综合性技术学科。其基本任务是将药物制成适合患者应用的最佳给药形式，是基础研究与临床应用的重要桥梁。药剂学实验作为重要的专业实践课程，对培养学生基本技能、科学思维和创新能力具有重要作用。

　　本实验教材是中山大学药剂学教学团队在多年实践教学经验基础上编写而成的，入选实验也都是经多年教学实验反复验证的。此外，结合高等医药院校对药学类实验教学新的发展要求，本实验教材在强调基础理论和基本技能的同时也注重学生创新思维的培养。

　　本教材的内容分为以下几部分：①药剂学实验课程要求与基本技能，包括药剂学实验室学生守则和实验中常见安全问题，同时列举实验报告的基本格式和撰写要求。②处方前研究，包括溶解度、油水分配系数、吸湿性、多晶型、酸度系数、流变性、粉体流动性、药物辅料相容性和药物渗透性等的常用测定方法，是研制安全、有效、稳定、可控的药物制剂的重要前提和必要保障。③普通制剂的制备，包括溶液型液体制剂、混悬剂、乳剂、注射剂、颗粒剂、硬胶囊剂、片剂、软膏剂、栓剂和涂膜剂的制备及质量评价，旨在理论与实践相结合帮助学生掌握重要剂型的制备方法与质量评价。④新剂型与新技术，包括固体分散体、包合物、微球、可溶性微针、吸入粉雾剂、骨架缓释片、微乳和固体脂质纳米粒的制备和评价，确保实验教学内容紧跟学科的发展，培养学生科学思维和创新能力。⑤附录，包括药剂学实验常用仪器使用说明以及部分质量评价方法，特别是仪器的正确使用，直接关系到实验的成败，成为基本技能的重要组成部分。

　　本实验教材主要供高等院校医药本科药学类专业的药剂学实验教学使用。由于本教材包括了处方前研究内容、常用仪器操作规范和质量评价手段，也可以作为医院药房、研究单位、工厂企业等从事药物制剂研究人员的参考用书。

　　本教材编写过程中得到邹祎晴、李彭宇、杨绚、牛博艺、马成、荣贺慧、熊梦婷和陈小楠等研究生的大力支持，中山大学 2017 级本科生亦对本教材的编写提出宝贵意见，在此一并表示感谢。

　　由于编者的水平有限，在实验内容编排和语言表达方面恐有欠妥之处，诚请广大读者批评指正，编者将不胜感激。

编　者

2020 年 6 月

目 录

第一部分 药剂学实验课程要求与基本技能

第一节 药剂学实验室学生守则

学生基本守则

（1）按时上课，非特殊原因不得申请调课及补课。

（2）提前 10 min 到达实验室，签到，穿着实验服，禁止长发披肩进入实验室。书包摆放至指定位置，保持桌面整洁。

（3）认真预习实验内容，包括实验中涉及的原理、操作、注意事项及预习思考等。课堂上会进行抽查提问或小测，成绩计入总评。

（4）实验过程中可以讨论，但禁止大声喧哗。

（5）原始记录真实、完整。发现篡改、伪造或抄袭他人数据或报告的，取消该次实验成绩。出现 2 次以上实验结果真实性问题的，本课程成绩总评以 0 分计。

（6）认真学习本教材第一部分"药剂学实验课程要求与基本技能"，规范实验操作，提高实验技能。

（7）本教材的药剂学实验是以剂型分类进行编写的，每个实验可能会包括若干个制剂，工作量大，实验过程中小组成员需进行相应分工，合理安排时间。

（8）养成良好的科研习惯，公用试剂用完后整理好并放回原处；爱护仪器，保持仪器的清洁。尤其是天平的使用，请根据试剂的质量选择适宜量程的天平，并注意挥发性、腐蚀性试剂的称量。

（9）实验过程中产生的垃圾应及时清理；针头和玻璃应扔进专用的回收箱；实验产生的废液应分类回收。

（10）做完实验后，关闭并清洁仪器，整理台面，锁好柜子，归还钥匙至指定位置，签名后方可离开。如实验中涉及水浴锅的使用，实验结束后应将水浴锅断电，并将其中的水放空。

（11）值日生做完清洁并关闭实验室的门窗水电，经老师检查合格后方可离开。

（12）熟悉实验室布局，明确救生通道、安全设施的位置。淋洗、冲眼、急救箱等安全设施安装在实验室门口，危急时可自行取用或救助他人。

第二节　药剂学实验室常见安全问题

一、常见安全问题

态度不端正、缺乏知识和错误操作等都可引发安全事故，进入实验室的每个人应时刻保持警惕。具体包括：

（1）实验中腐蚀性化学物品（如碘、甲酚、酸、碱等）腐蚀皮肤或衣物的事件时有发生，因此实验过程中应穿着实验服，禁止穿短裤、裙子和凉鞋等，防止皮肤暴露在外面。

（2）牢记实验室及配套实验区域的危险性标识。

（3）回收液体时应看清标签，分类回收。若将酸、碱废液混合可能导致废液桶爆炸。

（4）使用液体试剂时应小心，若发生倾洒应及时清理。避免溶剂洒在地上，导致人员摔跤；若洒在桌面上，没有及时清理，可能造成人员损伤。如甲酚洒在桌面上，可因接触而导致皮肤损伤；液体溅到插座上，可能造成漏电。

（5）使用离心机前应将离心管连同离心筒一起称量平衡。若质量不平衡或离心筒没有卡稳，在离心过程中可导致离心筒掉落而失衡。离心机失衡时应马上切断电源。

（6）使用通风橱进行各种操作前，应检查通风橱是否正常工作。

（7）进行流通蒸汽灭菌操作时应计时，避免锅中水烧干，导致安瓿接触炽热锅底，发生高温爆裂；进行安瓿瓶的熔封操作时应小心，避免烫伤；掰开安瓿瓶时，统一用砂盘划痕后掰开，以防手指被划破。

（8）在紫外灯下观察薄层色谱结果时应注意防护眼部，避免灼伤。

二、急救处理方法

（1）外伤处理：如被玻璃划伤后应及时检查体内有无玻璃碎屑残留，做好清理工作后，涂抹红药水进行止痛和消毒处理。

（2）烫伤和烧伤的急救处理：可先用无菌生理盐水冲洗，再用 1∶2 000 新洁尔灭冲洗，擦干伤口后用纱布包扎；对于电炉（汽）烫伤，可用泰国青草膏涂擦患处。

（3）化学灼伤：应迅速清理皮肤上的化学药品，并用大量的水冲洗，再用相应溶剂进行处理。碱类物质灼伤应采用 20 g/L 醋酸溶液清洗或直接扑以硼酸粉；酸液灼伤应采用饱和碳酸钠溶液进行冲洗。眼睛受到化学灼伤时，用冲眼仪的水流进行洗涤，但应避免水流直射眼球，更不要揉眼睛；碱灼伤可用 2% 硼酸淋洗，酸灼伤则用 2% 碳酸钠溶液淋洗。

（4）后处理：伤口在做初步急救处理后，应视情况决定是否送往医院进行进一步检查和治疗。

第三节　实验报告的基本格式

实验报告的基本格式范例

实验报告是科学研究活动中，实验人员通过实验观察、分析、综合与判断，如实地把实验的全过程和实验结果用文字或图表形式记录下来的书面材料。撰写实验报告是学生加深对知识的理解和认识，化被动学习为主动探索的过程。学生对于实验细节的记录，有利于日后随时查阅，并总结科学规律。常见的实验报告包括的内容见表 1-1。

表 1-1　实验报告格式范例

班级：_____	姓名：_____	学号：_____
	同组学生姓名：_____	学号：_____
日期：_____	温度：_____	湿度：_____
（一）实验名称		
（二）实验目的		
（三）实验原理		
（四）实验材料和仪器		
（五）实验内容		
（六）实验结果与讨论		
（七）思考题		
（八）建议		
（九）参考文献		

第四节　　实验报告的撰写

一、实验报告的内容基本要求

（1）真实，对实验的过程和结果如实记录，可以辅以图解帮助说明。

（2）完整，记录的现象和结果应是完整的，没有残缺的。

（3）准确，方法经得住重复和验证。

二、实验名称

实验名称应根据实验特点和需要，充分反映实验内容、实验目的或强调实验方法。一般按照教材的实验名称填写。

三、实验目的

实验目的应简明扼要地说明研究的意义及学习目标。

四、实验原理

实验原理应简要说明实验依据的理论，包括涉及的概念、定律和公式等，以及这些理论与本次实验之间的关联。

五、实验材料与仪器

应无遗漏地列出实验中用到的材料、试药与仪器。

六、实验内容

实验内容应包括所有的实验，重点介绍处方、工艺、质量检查及注意事项。对于实验中使用到的重要设备，可对其结构、操作及操作注意事项进行说明。

七、实验结果与讨论

实验结果与讨论是实验报告的主体，包括对实验现象的观察、记录、分析和讨论。

（一）观察与记录

明确观察目的与主要的观察对象。观察实验要仔细，要注重对本质现象（即揭示事物本质特征的现象）的观察。应将观察到的现象以及测得的数据进行整理并加以分析，以文字、照片或图表的方式表述。记录现象要准确、客观，表述要简洁明晰。实验报告中所用的原理和方法，要有依据，新方法要进行方法学验证。

1. 文字叙述

根据实验目的将原始资料系统化、条理化，用准确的专业术语客观地描述实验现象和结果。对于现象的描述，可根据时间段来描述，变化前、变化中及变化后；可对实验中物质的形态［包括物质的状态（气、液、固）、溶解、沉淀的析出、气泡、气味等］、外观（包括物质的颜色、烟、雾、浑浊等）以及能量（包括物质变化中发生的光、电、热、声、爆炸等）进行描述。描述时不能以结论代替现象，要科学规范准确地使用术语，切忌专业术语口语化以及混乱使用专业术语。

2. 图表描述

用表格或图的方式使实验结果更清晰、更具有可比性，如应用曲线图可以使指标的变化趋势形象生动、直观明了。

（二）分析与讨论

根据实验中观察的现象以及测得的数据等，结合理论加以分析，最后用简要、准确的语言进行概括，得出结论。须结合已报道的相关研究结果进行讨论。如果实验结果和预期的结果一致，它说明了什么？可以验证什么理论？实验结果有什么意义？若结果和预期的结果不一致，应找出原因。如果是因为方法表述不详细或不准确导致的，应对实验方法进行修正；如果方法的某一步很容易错误操作，应在注意事项中加以说明。讨论部分应反映理论—实践—理论的学习思考过程。也可介绍本实验相关研究的进展以及尚存在的问题。

八、思考题

实验教材中的或者上课老师布置的思考题，是对实验内容的必要延伸。学生应认真思考，查阅资料并仔细回答，以加深对实验及相关理论的理解。

九、建议

建议部分可针对实验中出现的问题，对实验或实验教学提出建设性的意见。

十、参考文献

实验报告中若引用文献的数据、观点或方法的，应将文献的作者、题目、出版日期、出版单位等以参考文献的形式列在实验报告的最后。

第二部分　处方前研究

第一节　溶　解　度

一、定义

溶解度（solubility）指在一定温度（气体在一定压力）下，一定量溶剂中，达到饱和状态时溶解的最大药量，是反映药物溶解性的重要指标。药品的近似溶解度常按表2-1划分：

表2-1　近似溶解度

近似溶解度	定义
极易溶解	溶质1 g（mL）能在不到1 mL的溶剂中溶解
易溶	溶质1 g（mL）能在1 mL至不到10 mL的溶剂中溶解
溶解	溶质1 g（mL）能在10 mL至不到30 mL的溶剂中溶解
略溶	溶质1 g（mL）能在30 mL至不到100 mL的溶剂中溶解
微溶	溶质1 g（mL）能在100 mL至不到1 000 mL的溶剂中溶解
极微溶解	溶质1 g（mL）能在1 000 mL至不到10 000 mL的溶剂中溶解
几乎不溶或不溶	溶质1 g（mL）在10 000 mL及以上体积的溶剂中不能完全溶解

在需要准确评价药物溶解性时，通常会测定药物的特性溶解度或平衡溶解度。特性溶解度（intrinsic solubility）是指药物不含任何杂质，在溶剂中不发生解离或缔合，也不发生相互作用时所形成的饱和溶液的浓度，是药物的重要物理参数之一。平衡溶解度（equilibrium solubility），也称为表观溶解度（apparent solubility），是指在溶剂中加入过量的药物，待药物溶解达到平衡后，药物在溶剂中的饱和浓度。由于受各种因素影响，工作中实际测定的药物溶解度多为平衡溶解度。

生物药剂学分类系统（biopharmaceutics classification system，BCS）按照药物溶解性

和肠道渗透性的差别，将药物分为四类（图2-1），BCS Ⅰ类，高溶解性—高渗透性；BCS Ⅱ类，低溶解性—高渗透性；BCS Ⅲ类，高溶解性—低渗透性；BCS Ⅳ类，低溶解性—低渗透性。不同国家/机构对高溶解性和高渗透性的定义不同，具体见表2-2。

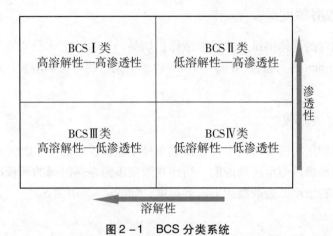

图2-1　BCS分类系统

表2-2　不同国家/机构高溶解性和渗透性的定义

国家/机构	高溶解性定义	高渗透性定义
FDA	单次给药的最大剂量能溶解在不超过250 mL的pH为1.0～7.5的37 ℃水溶液中	制剂口服后吸收程度不低于90%
EMA	单次给药的最大剂量能溶解在不超过250 mL的pH为1.0～6.8的37 ℃水溶液中（通常在3份pH为1.0、4.5、6.8的缓冲液中测定）	制剂口服后吸收程度不低于85%
WHO	单次给药的最大剂量能溶解在不超过250 mL的pH为1.2～6.8的37 ℃水溶液中	制剂口服后吸收程度不低于85%

二、意义

药物溶解度是制剂设计时首先需要掌握的重要信息，是决定药物能否设计成溶液型制剂的主要依据。药物溶解度与固体制剂的溶出速率呈现一定的相关性，并直接影响药物在体内的吸收和生物利用度。

BCS概念的提出最初是基于对药品上市后的变更以及放大给予免除生物等效性研究的考虑。近年来，基于BCS分类系统免除生物等效研究的应用已扩展至口服仿制药的申请。此外，以药物溶解性和渗透性为分类依据的BCS系统对候选药物的选择、药物剂型设计、固体制剂溶出度试验等方面均具有重要的指导意义。

三、测定方法

（一）近似溶解度

称取研成细粉的固体供试品或量取液体供试品，加入一定体积的溶剂中，在（25 ±
2）℃下，每隔 5 min 强力振摇 30 s。30 min 后，当无目视可见的溶质颗粒或液滴时，即
视为完全溶解。

（二）平衡溶解度

取过量的药物加入适量溶剂中，在恒温条件下振荡，每隔一定时间取样，样品经离
心或过滤并适当稀释后测定药物浓度。当药物浓度不随振荡时间的延长而增加，达到平
衡时，对应的药物浓度即为药物的平衡溶解度，如图 2 - 2 中的 S。

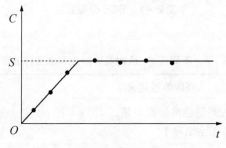

图 2 - 2　平衡溶解度测定曲线

（三）特性溶解度

特性溶解度根据相溶原理测定。在 N 份相同体积的溶剂中加入过量的药物，注意使
其过量程度呈现一个梯度，测定不同过量药物浑浊液的平衡溶解度。以药物质量与溶剂
体积的比为横坐标，相对应的平衡溶解度为纵坐标作图，将各个平衡溶解度拟合成直
线，将直线外推到纵坐标，直线与纵轴相交，交点所显示的溶解度即为特性溶解度 S_0
（图 2 -3）。

图 2 -3 中直线 1 显示在该溶液中药物发生解离，或者杂质或溶剂对药物有复合及
增溶作用等；直线 2 显示药物纯度高，无解离与缔合，无相互作用；直线 3 则显示发生
抑制溶解的同离子效应。

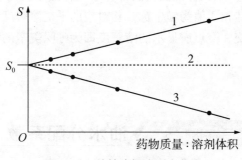

图2-3 特性溶解度测定曲线

注意事项

测定溶解度时，要注意恒温搅拌和平衡时间，注意取样温度与测定温度保持一致并滤除未溶解的药物。无论是测定平衡溶解度还是特性溶解度，一般都需要在室温（25℃）和体温（37℃）两种条件下进行，以便为药物使用、运输和贮存条件提供依据。

四、吲哚美辛特性溶解度与平衡溶解度的测定示例

（一）吲哚美辛在不同溶剂中的标准曲线的绘制

称取约10 mg吲哚美辛对照品，加1 mL无水乙醇溶解，再加入适量蒸馏水（或磷酸盐缓冲溶液）稀释、定容，得浓度约为20 μg/mL的吲哚美辛贮备液。精密量取不同体积的贮备液于25 mL容量瓶中，加入蒸馏水（或磷酸盐缓冲溶液）定容，摇匀，得到浓度为5～20 μg/mL的系列溶液。采用紫外分光光度计测定320 nm处的吸光度，以吲哚美辛浓度为横坐标，吸光度为纵坐标绘制标准曲线。

（二）吲哚美辛在不同介质中平衡溶解度的测定

配制pH分别为6.8、7.4和8.0的磷酸盐缓冲溶液。取以上3种缓冲液及蒸馏水，分别加入过量吲哚美辛，于37℃下恒温振摇至溶解平衡，随后5 000 r/min离心10 min，取上清液经0.45 μm微孔滤膜过滤，弃去初滤液，取续滤液稀释一定倍数后，采用紫外分光光度法测定320 nm处吸光度。采用标准曲线法计算药物在37℃下不同介质中的平衡溶解度。

（三）吲哚美辛特性溶解度的测定

分别称取约0.5 mg、1.0 mg、2.0 mg、4.0 mg、8.0 mg吲哚美辛加至15 mL具塞三角瓶中，加10 mL蒸馏水，于37℃下恒温振摇至溶解平衡，随后5 000 r/min离心10 min，取上清液经0.45 μm微孔滤膜过滤，续滤液稀释一定倍数，采用紫外分光光度

法测定 320 nm 处吸光度。采用标准曲线法计算不同样品中的药物浓度（平衡溶解度）。以吲哚美辛质量 – 溶剂体积比值为横坐标，相对应的平衡溶解度为纵坐标作图，拟合直线，外推直线与纵轴相交，交点所显示的溶解度即为吲哚美辛的特性溶解度。

第二节　油水分配系数

一、定义

油水分配系数（oil-water partition coefficiency，以 P 表示）是指当药物在水相和油相达到平衡时，药物在油相中的浓度和在水相中的浓度之比，通常以 $\lg P$ 表示。

二、意义

药物在体内的溶解、吸收、分布、转运与药物的水溶性和脂溶性有关，即和油水分配系数有关。一般而言，油水分配系数大小适中有利于药物穿膜转运和吸收。

体外测定油水分配系数，是为了模拟生物体内药物在水相和生物相之间的分配情况。由于正辛醇的溶解度参数与生物膜整体的溶解度参数相近，故正辛醇 – 水系统被广泛用于油水分配系统的测定。

三、测定方法

测量油水分配系数最常用的方法是摇瓶法，以正辛醇饱和的水为水相，水饱和的正辛醇为油相。称取一定量的药物溶解于水相或油相，然后把含药相与另一相按照 1∶1 的比例混合，在恒定温度下振摇至平衡，测定药物在两相中的浓度 $C_油$ 和 $C_水$，$C_油$ 与 $C_水$ 的比值即为油水分配系数。

四、布洛芬的油水分配系数测定示例

配制 pH 为 7.4 的磷酸盐缓冲溶液。分别取 100 mL 正辛醇与磷酸盐缓冲液在分液漏斗中混合，盖上盖子，静置 24 h 后，上层即为磷酸盐缓冲液饱和的正辛醇，下层即为正辛醇饱和的磷酸盐缓冲液。分别取上层和下层，备用。

精密称取布洛芬约 10 mg，用磷酸盐缓冲液饱和的正辛醇制备浓度约 50 μg/mL 的

贮备液（$C_总$），精密量取 20 mL 置三角瓶中。往三角瓶中加入 20 mL 正辛醇饱和的磷酸盐缓冲液，置于 37 ℃恒温振荡器中振荡 48 h，直至药物在两相中分配达到平衡。将两相转入分液漏斗中，静置 15 min 使分层，分离出水相，3 000 r/min 离心 10 min，收集水相，采用紫外分光光度法测定 263 nm 处的吸光度。建立布洛芬在正辛醇饱和的磷酸盐缓冲液中的标准曲线，根据标准曲线计算布洛芬在水相中的浓度 $C_水$，按照式（2-2-1）计算油水分配系数 P：

$$P = (C_总 - C_水)/C_水 \qquad (2-2-1)$$

第三节　吸湿性

一、定义

药物的吸湿性（hygroscopicity）是指在一定温度及湿度条件下，该物质吸收水分能力或程度的特性。根据药物吸湿特征的不同，常采用表 2-3 中的分类方式。

表2-3　吸湿性

吸湿性	定义
潮解	吸收足量水分形成液体
极具吸湿性	吸湿增重不小于 15%
有吸湿性	吸湿增重小于 15% 但不小于 2%
略有吸湿性	吸湿增重小于 2% 但不小于 0.2%
无或几乎无吸湿性	吸湿增重小于 0.2%

临界相对湿度（critical relative humidity，以 CRH 表示），是指水溶性药物在相对湿度增大到一定值时吸湿量急剧增加，一般把吸湿量开始急剧增加时的相对湿度称为临界相对湿度。CRH 为水溶性药物固有的特征参数，CRH 越大，越不易吸湿。

二、意义

将药物粉末置于湿度大于 CRH 的环境中容易发生不同程度的吸湿，致使粉末的流动性下降、固结、液化等，加快化学反应的发生从而降低药物稳定性。测定物料的 CRH 对防湿有重要意义，在药品的生产和贮藏过程中，应将环境相对湿度控制在物料 CRH 值以下，辅料也常用 CRH 值较大的物料。

三、测定方法

(一)吸湿率

取干燥的培养皿一套,精密称重(m_1)。取供试品适量,平铺于上述培养皿中,使供试品的厚度约为 1 mm,盖好皿盖,精密称重(m_2)。将培养皿敞口,并与皿盖同置于恒温恒湿条件下直至恒重(m_3),按照式(2-3-1)计算吸湿率:

$$吸湿率 = \frac{m_3 - m_2}{m_2 - m_1} \times 100\% \qquad (2-3-1)$$

辅料的使用有利于改变药物制剂的吸湿性。药物中加入不同种类的辅料,测定制剂的吸湿率,绘制吸湿曲线,可以考察不同辅料对于药物制剂吸湿性的影响。同理,也可考察不同比例辅料的联合应用对制剂吸湿性的影响。

(二)临界相对湿度

称取 6 份药物(粉末或颗粒),每份 1~2 g,置于盛有不同盐溶液的玻璃干燥器(不同相对湿度)中,于 25 ℃的恒温箱中保存 7 d,同上操作测定药物的吸湿率,以吸湿率为纵坐标,相对湿度为横坐标作图,对曲线两端作切线,两切线的交点对应的横坐标即为药物的 CRH。

四、水杨酸钠吸湿率与临界相对湿度的测定示例

(一)水杨酸钠吸湿率的测定

取水杨酸钠适量,置于干燥器中脱湿 12 h 以上至恒定质量,备用。将底部盛有过饱和氯化钠溶液的干燥器在 25 ℃放置 48 h,使其内部相对湿度约为 75%。取干燥的培养皿精密称取其质量(m_1),于培养皿中加入上述干燥的水杨酸钠约 2 g(平行 3 份),精密称量水杨酸钠与培养皿的总质量(m_2),然后敞口置于盛有过饱和氯化钠溶液的干燥器中,分别于 2 h、4 h、8 h、12 h、24 h、72 h、168 h、240 h 精密称量(m_3),计算吸湿率。

(二)水杨酸钠的临界相对湿度测定

配制醋酸钾、碳酸钾、硝酸镁、碘化钾、氯化钠、氯化钾和硝酸钾的饱和盐溶液,置于玻璃干燥器中,25 ℃放置 48 h,使相对湿度分别达到 23%、43%、55%、69%、75%、84% 和 92%。同上测定药物在不同相对湿度条件下的吸湿率,以吸湿率为纵坐标,相对湿度为横坐标作图,对曲线两端作切线,两切线的交点对应的横坐标即为水杨酸钠的 CRH。

第四节 ＼＼ 多 晶 型

一、定义

药物存在两种及两种以上的晶型（晶态物质晶格内分子的排列形式），称为多晶型（polymorphism），又称为同质多晶型现象。多晶型包括晶体状态和无定形状态，也包括溶剂化物和水化物。晶型受温度、光照、氧化、压力、湿度等因素影响。

二、意义

多晶型药物由于内部分子排列不同，很可能在外观、溶解度及溶解速率、熔点、稳定性、生物利用度及药效等方面存在明显差异。该现象在口服固体制剂方面表现尤为明显。因此，在对多晶型药物进行研发以及审评时，应对其晶型进行充分分析。

三、测定方法

多晶型的测定分为晶型种类的鉴别（定性）和晶型含量的测定（定量），以下仅介绍定性测定方法。

（一）绝对鉴别法

绝对鉴别法可独立完成晶型鉴别，此方法仅适用于晶型原料药。最常用的方法为单晶 X 射线衍射法，即通过测定供试品成分（化合物、结晶水或溶剂）、晶胞参数（a，b，c，α，β，γ）、分子对称性（晶系、空间群）、分子键合方式（氢键、盐键、配位键）、分子构象等参量变化，实现对固体晶型的鉴别。

（二）相对鉴别法

相对鉴别法指借助已知物质的晶型信息完成晶型种类鉴别的方法，该法适用于不同晶型药物的图谱数据间存在差异时的晶型种类鉴别。将测得的供试品晶型与已知晶型药物的图谱数据进行比对：当供试品化学物质确定且与已知晶型样品鉴别方法一致时，若测得的供试品图谱或数据与已知晶型样品不同，就说明供试品中的晶型种类或成分发生了改变，可能由一种晶型变为另外一种晶型，或混晶物质种类或比例发生了改变。

常用的方法包括粉末 X 射线衍射法、拉曼光谱法、红外光谱法、差式扫描量热法、偏光显微法等，其中，以下 3 种方法使用最为广泛。

1. 粉末 X 射线衍射法

通过检测供试品衍射峰的数量、位置（2θ 或 d）、强度（相对或绝对）以及各峰强度之比等参量变化，可鉴别晶型物质的状态。通常晶态物质粉末 X 射线图谱呈锐峰，无定型态物质粉末 X 射线图谱呈弥散峰。在判断晶态物质的晶体状态一致性时，应确保样品间的衍射峰数量相同，2θ 值衍射峰位置误差范围在 ±0.2° 内，相同位置衍射峰的相对峰强度误差在 ±5% 内且衍射峰的强弱顺序一致；在判断无定型态物质的晶体状态一致性时，应确保样品间的弥散衍射峰几何拓扑形状完全一致。

2. 拉曼光谱法

利用供试品中不同晶型物质特有的分子极化率变化引起指定波长范围内的拉曼光谱吸收峰的位置、强度、峰形几何拓扑等参量变化，实现对晶型物质状态的鉴别。

3. 红外光谱法

不同晶型药物分子振动时特有的偶极矩不同，与其对应的红外光谱吸收峰的位置、强度、峰形几何拓扑等参量也会出现差异，据此能实现对药物晶体状态的鉴别。该方法适用于分子作用力发生变化时的晶体状态的鉴别，一般采用衰减全反射进样法。制备样品时，应注意避免研磨与压片，以免由于制样操作引起样品的晶型转变。

第五节　酸 度 系 数

一、定义

酸度系数（acidity constant），又名酸离解常数，量符号为 pK_a，是酸解离平衡常数（K_a）的常用对数的相反数，其定义式为 $pK_a = -\lg K_a$。pK_a 的大小反映了酸的强度，pK_a 越低，酸性越强。

以一元弱酸（monprotic weak acid，HA）为例，其在水溶液中存在以下解离平衡：

$$HA + H_2O \rightleftharpoons H_3O^+ + A^-$$

其解离平衡常数表达式为

$$K_a = \frac{[H_3O^+][A^-]}{[HA]}$$

对上式等号两边取负对数，得式（2 - 5 - 1）：

$$pK_a = pH + \lg\frac{[HA]}{[A^-]} \tag{2-5-1}$$

在一定温度下，当 HA 溶液中 [A$^-$] = [HA] 时，pH 即为 pK_a。

二、意义

大多数药物为有机弱酸或有机弱碱。由于 pK_a 的不同，药物在不同 pH 介质中解离度不同。通常，解离型药物不易吸收，而非解离型药物则因较易通过细胞膜而容易被吸收。

三、测定方法

弱酸或弱碱性药物的 pK_a 常用滴定法测定。对于一元酸的 pK_a 测定，可用碱溶液（如氢氧化钠溶液）滴定，以碱溶液的体积为横坐标，滴定溶液的 pH 为纵坐标，绘制滴定曲线。注意，当滴入一半体积的碱溶液后，溶液中 [A$^-$] = [HA]，即 $\lg \dfrac{[HA]}{[A^-]} = 0$，此时的溶液的 pH = p$K_a$。多元酸在水中是逐级解离的，具有多个 p$K_a$，可通过分步滴定法滴定。

当药物具有紫外吸收，且分子型（HA）、离子型（A$^-$）药物的紫外吸收光谱有显著差异时，可采用分光光度法测定其 pK_a，即取待测药物配制成 3 份浓度相等的溶液，分别编号为 1、2、3 号。通过调节 pH，使 1 号溶液中药物部分为 HA，部分为 A$^-$；2 号溶液中药物全部以 HA 形式存在；3 号溶液中药物全部以 A$^-$ 的形式存在。在一定波长处分别测定 1、2、3 号溶液的吸收度 A、A_{HA}、A_A，按照式（2-5-2）计算药物的 pK_a：

$$pK_a = pH + \lg \frac{A - A_A}{A_{HA} - A} \qquad (2-5-2)$$

式中，pH 为溶液 1 的 pH。

第六节 流 变 性

一、定义

在适当外力的作用下，物质所具有的流动性和变形性称为流变性（rheological property）。流体的剪切速率（rate of sheer）和剪切应力（shearing stress）的关系可反映其流变学性质，根据二者的变化关系可将流体分为牛顿流体（或理想流体）和非牛顿流体。

在没有屈服力的情况下，牛顿流体的剪切应力和剪切速率呈线性变化，水、空气、油、液状石蜡及低分子化合物的纯液体稀溶液或高分子稀溶液均属于此类。非牛顿流体的剪切应力和剪切速率呈非线性变化，高分子的浓溶液、胶体溶液、混悬液、乳剂和软膏剂均属于此类。

二、意义

引用流变学理论可对乳剂、混悬剂、半固体制剂等的剂型设计、处方组成、质量控制等进行评价。理想的混悬剂应该在贮藏过程中保持较高的黏度，而在振摇、倒出、铺展时能自由流动。优良的乳剂应该在静止时保持较高的黏度，以保持体系稳定，当振摇和倾倒时黏度降低，利于倒出。

半固体制剂，如软膏剂、凝胶剂、糊剂等，其流变学特征可指导处方设计和质量评价。软膏剂与凝胶剂的可挤出性直接影响患者用药的依从性。药品在开盖时不应自动流出，当挤压时应缓慢挤出，停止挤压则不流出。皮肤使用的半固体制剂，可以通过添加具有触变性的基质调节药品的黏度，给力时可使药品容易涂展，停止给力时药物黏附于皮肤。眼部给药的触变性原位凝胶给药系统可在滴入眼部时发生相转变，形成具有黏弹性的凝胶，以提高其在眼部的滞留时间。

三、测定方法

流变性质的测定原理是求出物体流动的速度和引起流动所需的力之间的关系。最常测定的流变学性质是黏度（viscosity）和稠度（consistency）。黏度指流体对流动产生阻抗能力的性质；稠度指流体在规定的剪切力或剪切速度下变形的程度。

（一）黏度的测定

黏度的表示方法包括动力黏度、运动黏度或特性黏度。黏度的测量方法包括平氏毛细管黏度计、乌氏毛细管黏度计和旋转黏度计等。其中，毛细管黏度计适用于牛顿流体运动黏度的测定，旋转黏度计适用于牛顿流体或非牛顿流体动力黏度的测定。此处仅介绍旋转黏度计测定法（参照《中国药典》2020 版通则 0633 黏度测定法）。

旋转黏度计法：以转子型旋转黏度计（图 2-4）为例，通过将某些类型的转子浸入待测样品中，并以恒定的角速度（ω）转动，测定马达转动产生的扭矩（M），根据公式 $\eta = K\dfrac{M}{\omega}$ 计算待测样品的黏度。通常情况下，转子型黏度计常数 K 是通过采用标准黏度液校准得到，故其测定结果为相对黏度。

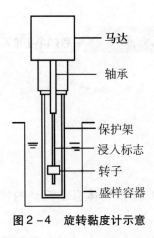

图2-4 旋转黏度计示意

（二）稠度的测定

软膏、乳膏等半固体制剂的稠度可用插度计进行测定。如图2-5所示，在一定温度下，将插度计中质量为150 g的金属锥体的锥尖放在供试品表面，以插入的深度评定供试品的稠度，以0.1 mm为1个单位，称为插入度。测定时需将待测样品熔化倒入适宜大小的容器中，静置使样品凝固且表面尽量光滑，保持样品内温度为均匀的25 ℃，并调节插度计底座水平。一般稠度大的样品插入度小，稠度小的样品插入度大。合格软膏剂的插入度通常规定在200～300个单位范围内。

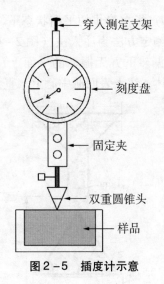

图2-5 插度计示意

第七节 粉体流动性

一、定义

粉体的流动性（flowability）是指粉体自由流动的性能，其与粒子的形状、大小、表面状态、密度、空隙率等有关。

二、意义

颗粒剂、胶囊剂、片剂等多种制剂的制备过程均涉及多种流动现象，因此，粉体的流动性对制剂质量，如重量差异、装量差异及含量均匀度等有较大影响。

三、测定方法

（一）休止角

休止角（angle of repose，θ）指在静止的平衡状态下，粉体堆积层的自由斜面与水平面所形成的最大角。常用的测定方法为注入法（图2-6），即将漏斗悬于铁架台上，表面皿倒扣（皿口朝下）置于漏斗下方无振动的平面上，调整表面皿使其原点与漏斗呈垂直线。从漏斗缓缓加入粉体，注入表面皿中心上，直到粉体堆积层斜边的物料沿圆

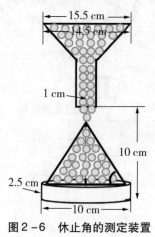

图2-6 休止角的测定装置

盘边缘自动流出，形成规则的圆锥体时停止注入。按照式（2-7-1）计算粉体的休止角：

$$\tan \theta = \frac{h}{r} \qquad\qquad (2-7-1)$$

式中，h 为圆锥体高度，r 为圆锥体半径。

休止角是检验粉体流动性好坏的最简便方法。休止角越小，粒子间摩擦力越小，流动性越好。一般认为 $\theta \leqslant 30°$ 时流动性好，$\theta \leqslant 40°$ 时可满足生产过程中对流动性的需求。

（二）流出速度

流出速度（flow velocity）指单位时间内从容器的小孔中流出粉体的量，如测定100 g 粉末流出小孔所需要的时间或测定 10 s 内流出小孔的样品量。流出速度的测定装置如图 2-7 所示，上方漏斗用于装样，测量粉末在下方漏斗流出的时间。若粉体不能流出，可加入直径为 100 μm 的玻璃球助流，测定粉体开始自由流动时所需玻璃球的最少量（即重量百分比，用 wt% 表示），以表示流动性。玻璃球加入量越多表明粉体流动性越差。

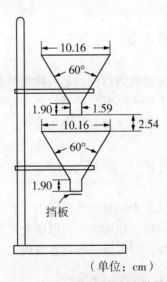

（单位：cm）

图 2-7　流出速度的测定装置

（三）压缩度

在无任何振动的条件下，将一定量的粉体填充至量筒中，振动量筒使粉体处于最紧状态，其振动后的最终体积 h_f 与初始体积 h_0 之差占初始体积的分数称为压缩度（compressibility index）。压缩度的测定常采用轻敲法（tapping method），如图 2-8 所示，将一定量的粉体轻轻装入量筒后测量初始体积，轻敲若干次使粉体处于最紧状态，然后再测量其最终体积。根据式（2-7-2）计算压缩度 C。一般来说，压缩度 20% 以下，表明该粉体的流动性较好。

$$C = \frac{h_0 - h_f}{h_0} \times 100\% \qquad\qquad (2-7-2)$$

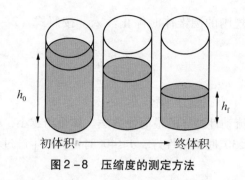

图 2-8　压缩度的测定方法

第八节　　药物辅料相容性

一、辅料选择的一般原则

辅料是制剂中除主药外其他物料的总称，是药物制剂的重要组成部分。辅料可根据药物和剂型的特点进行选择。生产药品所需的辅料必须符合药用标准，不应与主药发生不良相互作用，不影响制剂的含量测定及有关物质检查。

二、相容性研究的目的与意义

药物与辅料相容性研究为处方中辅料的选择提供了有益的信息和参考。可通过前期调研，了解辅料与辅料及药物间相互作用情况，以避免处方设计时选择不宜的辅料。对于缺乏相关研究数据辅料的选择，可考虑进行相容性研究。

三、药物与辅料相容性实验

药物与辅料的相容性实验没有统一的规定。目前常用基于药物理化性质的特点而设计的研究方法，同时进行分析方法的验证。例如口服固体制剂，可选若干种辅料，若辅料用量较大（如稀释剂等），可按主药∶辅料 = 1∶5 的比例混合；若辅料用量较小（如润滑剂等），可按主药∶辅料 = 20∶1 的比例混合。取一定量药物与辅料混合物，参照药物稳定性指导原则中影响因素实验方法或其他适宜的实验方法，重点考察性状、含量、有关物质等，从而判断辅料的加入对药物是否有影响。实验中宜用原料药和辅料分别做平行对照实验，以判别该变化是源于原料药本身还是辅料的加入。药物与辅料的相容性，常采用高温、高湿和强光实验进行测定。

（一）高温实验

将药物辅料混合物（粉末）置于敞口洁净干燥容器中，摊成约 5 mm 厚的薄层，于 60 ℃ 条件下放置 10 d，分别于第 0、5、10 d 取样，按稳定性实验重点考察项目进行测定。

（二）高湿实验

将药物辅料混合物（粉末）置于敞口洁净干燥容器中，摊成约 5 mm 厚的薄层，于 25 ℃、相对湿度（relative humidity，RH）为（90±5）% 的恒湿密闭容器中放置 10 d，分别于第 0、5、10 d 取样，按稳定性实验重点考察项目进行测定，并测定吸湿率。若吸湿率大于 5%，则在相对湿度（75±5）% 条件下，同法进行实验。

（三）强光实验

将药物辅料混合物样品粉末置于敞口洁净干燥容器中，摊成约 5 mm 厚的薄层，在药品强光照射实验箱内，照度（4 500±500）lx 条件下放置 10 天，分别于第 0、5、10 d 取样，按稳定性实验重点考察项目进行测定。

四、阿司匹林片的辅料相容性实验示例

以阿司匹林片为例，进行辅料相容性实验。阿司匹林片剂中常见辅料包括淀粉、酒石酸、淀粉浆及滑石粉等。将阿司匹林原料药与各辅料按表 2-4 至表 2-6 进行混合，取混合物适量，分别按高温、高湿及强光实验方法进行稳定性考察，采用高效液相色谱法测定阿司匹林含量与有关物质，考察各辅料与阿司匹林的相容性。

色谱条件：以十八烷基硅烷键合硅胶为填充剂；以乙腈 - 四氢呋喃 - 冰醋酸 - 水（20:5:5:70）为流动相；检测波长为 276 nm。理论塔板数按阿司匹林峰计算不低于 3 000，阿司匹林与水杨酸的分离度应符合要求。

表 2-4 阿司匹林片剂常用辅料相容性高温实验

项目	比例	高温实验（60 ℃）								
		第 0 天			第 5 天			第 10 天		
		性状	含量/%	有关物质	性状	含量/%	有关物质	性状	含量/%	有关物质
阿司匹林：淀粉	1:5									
阿司匹林：酒石酸	100:1									
阿司匹林：淀粉浆	3:1									
阿司匹林：滑石粉	20:1									

表2-5   阿司匹林片剂常用辅料相容性高湿实验

项目	比例	高湿实验（25 ℃，90%）								
		第0天			第5天			第10天		
		性状	含量/%	有关物质	性状	含量/%	有关物质	性状	含量/%	有关物质
阿司匹林：淀粉	1：5									
阿司匹林：酒石酸	100：1									
阿司匹林：淀粉浆	3：1									
阿司匹林：滑石粉	20：1									

表2-6   阿司匹林片剂常用辅料相容性强光实验

项目	比例	强光实验（4 500 lx）								
		第0天			第5天			第10天		
		性状	含量/%	有关物质	性状	含量/%	有关物质	性状	含量/%	有关物质
阿司匹林：淀粉	1：5									
阿司匹林：酒石酸	100：1									
阿司匹林：淀粉浆	3：1									
阿司匹林：滑石粉	20：1									

第九节　药物渗透性

一、意义

药物渗透性可以反映药物在人体内的吸收程度。对药物的渗透性进行测定，可以预测药物在体内的吸收，为药物制剂的开发提供参考。

二、测定方法

（一）人体内的药代动力学研究

人体内的药代动力学测定方法有质量平衡法和以静脉给药为对照的绝对生物利用度法。药物渗透性的判断，可根据质量平衡原理确定吸收程度（例如尿液中药物的回收率大于90%，或由代谢物的量换算成原形药物量大于90%）；或与静脉给药比较，若绝对生物利用度大于90%，可判断该药物为高渗透性药物。

（二）在体肠灌流法

在体肠灌流法包括在体单向肠灌流法、Doluisio 闭环肠灌流法等。其中，在体单向肠灌流法是指量取麻醉动物（通常是大鼠）一定长度的肠段，两端插管，将药液用恒速泵灌流肠腔，每隔一定时间收集出口管中灌流液，测定药物浓度的方法。

（三）离体肠囊法

离体肠囊法包括外翻肠囊法、未外翻肠囊法及尤斯灌流模型法等。其中，外翻肠囊法是指取一定长度的肠段一端结扎，并翻转肠段使肠黏膜层在外、浆膜层在内，缓冲液冲洗后结扎另一端，形成肠囊，向肠囊内注入空白缓冲液（受体侧），然后将肠囊置于含药缓冲液中（供体侧），整个装置通入碳合气（95% O_2，5% CO_2），置于 37 ℃恒温水浴中，定时从肠囊内取样检测药物浓度，实验结束后测量肠囊内表面积。

若采用以上两种渗透性测定方法，则可根据式（2-9-1）计算小肠有效渗透率 P_{eff}（effective permeability）来进行渗透性判断：

$$P_{eff} = Q_{in}(C_{in} - C_{out})/2\pi rLC_{out} \qquad (2-9-1)$$

其中，Q_{in} 为流速；C_{in} 和 C_{out} 分别为灌入液与流出液中的药物浓度；r 为半径；L 为空肠段长度。常将 $P_{eff} > 2 \times 10^{-4}$ cm/s 作为高渗透性的下限。

（四）体外细胞模型法

体外细胞模型法是指通过培养人结肠癌细胞上皮细胞（human colon carcinoma cell line，Caco-2）在 Transwell 孔板中得到单层细胞模型，开展研究时，将药物添加到细胞单层的一侧。孵育一定的时间后，测定另一侧的药物浓度，并计算药物的渗透速率。

注意事项

考虑到药物在透过胃肠壁膜前可能会有部分降解，为证明药物从胃肠道消除是由于药物透过胃肠壁膜而不是发生降解，研究中需注意考察药物在胃肠道中的稳定性。

对于前体药物，其渗透性的测定取决于前体药物向活性药物转化的机制和部位。若前药在透过肠壁膜后才转化为活性药物，则需测定前药的渗透性；若前药在胃肠道内已转化为活性药物，则应测定活性药物的渗透性。

三、常用模型药物

在药物渗透性研究时，常使用模型药物做比较。用于体内、外吸收研究的有关模型药物见表2 -7。

表2 -7　用于药物渗透性分类研究的几种模型药物

药物	渗透性类别	评价
α - 甲基多巴	低	氨基酸转运模型药物
安替比林	高	渗透性标示物
阿替洛尔	低	细胞间转运模型药物
甘露醇	高或低	渗透性高到低的边缘模型药物
美托洛尔	高或低	渗透性高到低的边缘模型药物
PEG400 - 4000	低	体内研究中不被吸收的模型药物
维拉帕米	高	体外研究中 P-gp 外排转运的阳性模型药物

参考文献

[1] 国家药典委员会. 中华人民共和国药典 [M]. 北京：中国医药科技出版社，2020.

[2] 方亮. 药剂学 [M]. 8 版. 北京：人民卫生出版社，2016.

[3] 崔福德. 药剂学实验指导 [M]. 3 版. 北京：人民卫生出版社，2011.

[4] 晁若冰，伍朝赟，贺晓英. 弱酸弱碱性药物 pK_a 值的分光光度测定法 [J]. 华西药学杂志，1990，5 (2)：104 - 106.

[5] 曹筱琛，贾飞，陶巧凤. 药物与辅料相容性研究进展 [J]. 中国现代应用药学，2013，30 (2)：223 - 228.

第三部分　普通制剂的制备

实验一　溶液型液体制剂的制备

一、实验目的

（1）掌握溶液型液体制剂的制备方法。
（2）掌握增溶与助溶在液体制剂制备中的作用。

二、实验原理

液体制剂（liquid pharmaceutical preparations）是指药物分散在适宜的分散介质中制成的可供内服或外用的液体形态的制剂。液体制剂根据分散状态的不同可分为溶液型、乳浊型和混悬型。溶液型液体制剂为澄明液体，溶液中药物分散度大，吸收较快。溶液型液体制剂又可分为低分子溶液剂和高分子溶液剂。常用的分散介质为水、乙醇、丙二醇、甘油、聚乙二醇或油等。

低分子溶液剂系指小分子药物以分子或离子状态分散在溶剂中形成的可供内服或外用的均相液体制剂。高分子溶液剂系指高分子化合物溶解于溶剂中制成的均相液体制剂，其中，以水为溶剂的称为亲水性高分子溶液剂或称胶浆剂，以非水溶剂制备的称为非水性高分子溶液剂。低分子溶液剂和高分子溶液剂均属于热力学稳定系统。

低分子溶液型液体制剂的制备方法主要有溶解法、稀释法和化学反应法，其中，溶解法最为常用。高分子溶液的形成则需要经历有限溶胀和无限溶胀两个过程。首先将高分子化合物分次撒在水面上或将其黏附于已润湿的器壁上以增加水与高分子材料的接触面积。然后，水分子渗入高分子化合物的分子间空隙中并与其亲水基团发生水化作用而使之体积膨胀，最后高分子空隙间充满了水分子，该过程称有限溶胀。由于高分子空隙间存在的水分子降低了高分子之间的分子间作用力，故溶胀过程继续进行，最终高分子化合物完全分散在水中形成高分子溶液，这一过程称为无限溶胀。无限溶胀过程可采取搅拌或加热等方法加速完成。

根据液体制剂制备的需要可加入助溶剂、增溶剂、潜溶剂、抗氧剂、矫味剂、着色剂等附加剂。

增溶与助溶是药剂学中增加难溶性药物溶解度的常用方法。增溶（solubilization）系指难溶性药物在表面活性剂溶液中溶解度增大并形成澄明溶液的过程。表面活性剂通常在临界胶束浓度以上才发挥增溶作用。具有增溶能力的表面活性剂称增溶剂（solubilizer），被增溶的物质称为增溶质（solubilizates）。药物的增溶作用受诸多因素影响，如增溶剂和增溶质的性质、增溶温度、增溶质的加入顺序等。本实验中甲酚皂溶液是钠肥皂形成胶团使微溶于水的甲酚增溶制得，甲酚在钠肥皂中可增溶至50%的浓度。助溶（hydrotropy）系指难溶性药物与加入的第三种物质在溶剂中形成可溶性络合物、复盐或缔合物，以增加药物在溶剂中的溶解度。这第三种物质称为助溶剂。助溶剂可溶于水，多为低分子化合物，常分为两大类：一类是某些有机酸及其钠盐，如苯甲酸钠、水杨酸钠和对氨基苯甲酸等；另一类是酰胺类化合物，如尿素和烟酰胺等。助溶机制较复杂，许多机理至今尚未清楚。一般根据药物的性质选用与之能形成水溶性分子间络合物、复盐或缔合物的物质。本实验中碘化钾为助溶剂。

溶液剂的质量检查一般包括外观、色泽、pH及含量测定等。

三、预习思考

（1）简述助溶剂和增溶剂的主要区别。

（2）如何在实验操作过程中减少甲酚的挥发，从而降低空气中甲酚浓度升高导致的黏膜刺激性？

（3）高分子溶解可分为哪两个阶段？简述高分子溶液的制备过程。

四、实验材料与仪器

1. 实验药剂

碘、碘化钾、甲酚、氢氧化钠、植物油、软皂、乙醇、薄荷脑、冰片、卡波姆940、丙三醇、香精、色素、三乙醇胺、吐温80、革兰氏染色试剂盒、蒸馏水。

2. 实验仪器

恒温水浴箱、pH试纸、研钵、天平、烧杯、量筒、玻璃棒、容量瓶、光学显微镜。

五、实验内容

(一)复方碘溶液

1. 处方

碘	1. 25 g
碘化钾	2. 50 g
蒸馏水加至	25 mL

2. 实验步骤

取碘化钾置烧杯中,加入少量水,使完全溶解(接近碘化钾饱和溶液)。加入碘,搅拌使溶解。待碘充分溶解后,加水定容到 25 mL,观察其外观性状。

注意事项

(1)碘具有腐蚀性,称量时可用玻璃皿或蜡纸,不宜用纸,操作时应避免与皮肤或黏膜接触。

(2)制备时,预先将碘化钾加适量蒸馏水配成近饱和溶液,然后加入碘使其完全溶解后,方可加水稀释。

(3)碘溶液具有氧化性,应储存于密闭玻璃瓶内,不能直接与木塞、橡胶塞及金属塞接触。

(4)碘溶液易挥发,宜保存在棕色瓶子里,避免阳光照射。

(二)甲酚皂溶液

1. 处方

	处方 I	处方 II
甲酚	10 mL	10 mL
植物油	3. 46 g	—
氢氧化钠	0. 54 g	—
软皂	—	10 g
蒸馏水加至	50 mL	50 mL

2. 实验步骤

(1)处方 I:取氢氧化钠加水 2 mL,搅拌使其溶解,冷却至室温,将其加入植物油中,90 ℃水浴加热,时时搅拌。待 50%～70% 的溶液转变为絮状物时加入 1 mL 无水乙醇，稍加搅拌，放冷至室温。20 min 后重置水浴上加热，5 min 后进行搅拌，待物料黏稠度增加时加入 1 mL 无水乙醇，时时搅拌，直至皂化完全（半固体状）。若皂化不完全，可再添加 1 mL 无水乙醇搅拌至皂化完全。趁热加入甲酚，使溶解完全，放冷，加蒸馏水至 50 mL，混匀，即得。

（2）处方Ⅱ：取 10 g 市售软皂剪碎，加入 10 mL 甲酚中，搅拌使分散均匀，添加蒸馏水至 50 mL，搅拌均匀，即得。

（3）稀释试验：分别取处方Ⅰ和处方Ⅱ制得的甲酚皂各 1 mL，加蒸馏水稀释，观察稀释 2～20 倍以及超过 200 倍时溶液的澄清度。

注意事项

（1）甲酚与苯酚结构性质相似，但较苯酚的杀菌力强，在较高浓度时对皮肤有刺激性，宜小心操作；当空气中甲酚浓度较高时，对黏膜有一定的刺激性。

（2）甲酚在水中溶解度小（1∶50），植物油与氢氧化钠反应生成肥皂，利用肥皂的增溶作用，可制成纯度高达 50% 的甲酚皂溶液。本实验制备的是浓度为 20% 的甲酚皂溶液。

（3）皂化程度完全与否与成品质量密切相关，皂化速度可因加少量乙醇而加快，待反应完全后再加热除去乙醇。

（4）完全皂化的判断标准：产物为半固体，表面无明显油滴或油状物；或取少量产物，加约 10 倍量的水，振摇分散，应无油滴。

（5）甲酚务必趁热加入新生皂中，快速搅拌使其溶解（此过程在通风橱中操作），并快速转移至容量瓶中密闭，避免甲酚挥发至空气中造成污染。

（6）甲酚、肥皂、水三组分形成的溶液是一种复杂体系，具有胶体溶液的特性。上述三组分配伍比例适当为澄清溶液，且用水稀释时亦不混浊。

（三）花露水

1. 处方

薄荷脑	0.2 g
冰片	0.2 g
香精	1.0 g
色素	适量
无水乙醇	70 mL
蒸馏水加至	100 mL

2. 实验步骤

薄荷脑和冰片用少量无水乙醇溶解，加入香精和色素搅拌使其溶解。再加入剩余的无水乙醇搅拌均匀，蒸馏水加至 100 mL，室温下放置 1 周陈化，分装即得。

注意事项

（1）薄荷脑和冰片易溶于无水乙醇，微溶于水，应先用无水乙醇溶解后再加入蒸馏水。

（2）陈化是将薄荷脑、冰片与乙醇静置一段时间，使其充分反应，生成具有香味的脂肪酸酯，使溶液香味更加浓郁，掩盖并淡化乙醇原有的刺激性气味，也可减少香精的添加量。

（四）免洗洗手液

1. 处方

乙醇	65 mL
卡波姆 940	0.4 g
丙三醇	5.0 g
香精	1.0 g
色素	适量
三乙醇胺	适量
蒸馏水加至	100 g

2. 实验步骤

（1）洗手液的配制。取 25 mL 水，将卡波姆 940 均匀撒在水面上形成薄层，静置，待其完全溶胀（形成近似透明凝胶）后搅拌均匀，依次加入乙醇、丙三醇，混匀，再加入香精和适量色素搅拌均匀。最后滴加三乙醇胺（5～6 滴）调节 pH 为 7.0，蒸馏水加至 100 g，即得。

（2）抑菌效果评价。取清洁载玻片，在载玻片左右两侧各滴 1 滴蒸馏水，将清洁棉签用灭菌水润湿，在受试者左手 5 个手指上依次涂抹 2 次，然后将棉签上收集的细菌转移至载玻片左侧的水滴中。然后受试者取硬币大小的洗手液涂抹在手部，反复搓揉，使洗手液在手上分布均匀，特别注意搓揉手指与手掌，使其与洗手液充分接触。1 min 后取清洁棉签用灭菌水润湿，在受试者左手的 5 个手指上依次涂抹 2 次，然后将棉签上收集的细菌转移至载玻片右侧的水滴中，固定并进行革兰氏染色（方法详见附录ⅢA），在显微镜下观察洗手液使用前后微生物数量与种类的变化。

注意事项

卡波姆溶胀速度较慢，尽量将其撒在较大面积的水面上，铺成薄层，以加快有限溶胀过程。

六、实验结果与讨论

（1）描述复方碘溶液的外观性状。

（2）观察甲酚皂溶液处方 I 和处方 II 的外观以及以任意比例稀释的澄清度。

甲酚皂溶液的性状比较见表 3 – 1。

表 3 – 1　甲酚皂溶液的性状比较

处方	处方 I	处方 II
甲酚皂溶液		
稀释 2 倍		
稀释 20 倍		
稀释超过 200 倍		

（3）抑菌实验。用光学显微镜观察使用免洗洗手液前后受试者手上的细菌数，评价洗手液抑菌效果。

七、思考题

（1）写出甲酚皂实验中皂化反应方程式。加速皂化反应的方法有哪些？分析本实验中乙醇的作用。

（2）观察甲酚皂稀释 2～20 倍时溶液的澄清度的什么临床意义。

（3）花露水处方中的薄荷脑和冰片有什么药理作用？配制时有哪些注意事项？

Experiment 1　Preparation of Solutions

I . Purpose

（1）To master the conventional preparation methods of solutions.

（2）To master the roles of solubilization and hydrotropy in the preparation of solutions.

II . Principles

Liquid preparations are those in which the drugs are dispersed in a suitable dispersion medium in the form of liquid for internal or external use. Liquid preparations can be classified into solutions, emulsions and suspensions depending on the dispersion states. Among them, the solutions are transparent liquid, in which drugs have high dispersion degree and are absorbed quickly, and can be further divided into low molecular solutions and polymer solutions. Water, ethanol, propylene glycol, glycerin, polyethylene glycol or oil are commonly used dispersion media.

Low molecular solutions refer to homogeneous liquid preparation for internal or external use, and small molecule drugs are dispersed in dispersion solvent in molecular or ionic state. Polymer solutions are homogeneous liquid preparations prepared by dissolving polymer compounds in solvents. Among them, those using water as solvent are called hydrophilic polymer solutions or hydro gels. Polymer solutions prepared with non-aqueous solvent are called non-aqueous polymer solutions. Both low molecular solutions and polymer solutions are thermodynamically stable systems.

The preparation methods of low molecular solutions mainly include dissolution, dilution, and chemical reaction. Among them, the dissolution is the most commonly used. The formation of polymer solutions requires two processes: limited swelling and infinite swelling. Firstly, polymer compounds are sprinkled on the surface of water or pre-adhered it to wetted walls to increase the contact area between water and polymer materials. Subsequently, water molecules penetrate into the voids of polymer compounds and hydrate with the hydrophilic groups of polymer molecules to expand the volume, and finally the polymer voids are filled fully with water molecules. This process is called limited swelling. Water molecules existing between polymer voids remarkably reduce the intermolecular forces of polymer molecules, and the swelling process continues. Finally, polymer molecules are completely dispersed in water to form polymer solutions, and this procedure is called infinite swelling. The infinite swelling process can be accelerated by stirring or heating.

Hydrotropy agents, solubilizers, cosolvents, antioxidants, flavoring agents, coloring agents and other additives can be added according to the needs.

Solubilization and hydrotropy are common methods used to increase the solubility of poorly soluble drugs in pharmaceutics. Solubilization refers to the process of increasing the solubility of poorly soluble drugs by adding surfactants above the critical micelle concentration of surfactants. Here, the surfactants with solubilizing ability are called solubilizers, and the substances to be solubilized are called solubilizates. The solubilization of drugs is affected by many factors, such as the characteristics of solubilizers and solubilizates, temperature, the order of solubilizates addition. In this experiment, cresol is solubilized by sodium soap to form a micelle in which the concentration of cresol can be solubilized by 50%. Hydrotropy refers to adding the third substance to the system, mostly low molecule compounds, to form soluble complexes, double salts or association complex in a solvent with poorly soluble drugs and thus increasing the solubility of drugs in solvent. The third substance is called hydrotropy agent. The hydrotropy agents, soluble in water, are often divided into two categories: one is some organic acids and their sodium salts, such as sodium benzoate, sodium salicylate and p-aminobenzoic acid; the other is amide compounds, such as urea and nicotinamide. The solubilization mechanism of hydrotropy agents is complicated and unclear. Generally, the substances which can form water-soluble molecular complexes, double salts or associated matters with drugs are given a priority.

Quality inspections of solutions generally include appearance, color, pH and content determination.

III. Preview

(1) Briefly describe the main differences between hydrotropy agents and solubilizers.

(2) How to attenuate the evaporation of cresol to the air and thus reduce the irritation of cresol to mucosa membranes?

(3) What are the two phases of polymer dissolving? Briefly describe the preparation process of polymer solutions.

IV. Experiment materials and equipments

1. Reagents and experimental materials

Iodine, potassium iodide, cresol, sodium hydroxide, vegetable oil, soft soap, ethanol, menthol, borneol, carbomer 940, glycerol, fragrance, pigment, Trolamine, Tween-80, Gram staining kit, distilled water.

2. Experimental equipments

Constant temperature water bath, pH test strips, mortar, balance, beaker, graduated cylinder, glass rod, volumetric flask, optical microscope.

V. Experiment contents

1. Preparation of compound iodine solution

(1) Prescription:

Iodine	1.25 g
Potassium iodide	2.50 g
Distilled water added to	25 mL

(2) Procedures: Place potassium iodide in a beaker and add distilled water to make it dissolve completely to a high concentration (Near saturated solution of potassium iodide). Then add iodine to the solution and stir, making it dissolve completely. Finally, add distilled water to the whole volume of 25 mL and observe its appearance.

[Precautions]

(1) Iodine is corrosive. Glass or wax paper is used for weighing. It is not suitable to use common paper. Prevent skin and mucous membrane from iodine during the whole operation.

(2) Potassium iodide is dissolved by adding an appropriate amount of distilled water to form a near-saturated solution. When iodine completely dissolved, water is added to the whole volume.

（3）The compound iodine solution is a strong oxidant and therefore would be conserved in an airtight glass bottle. Avoid directly contact it with corks, rubber stoppers and metal plugs.

2. Preparation of cresol soap solution

（1）Prescription:

	Prescription I	Prescription II
Cresol	10 mL	10 mL
Vegetable oil	3.46 g	—
Sodium hydroxide	0.54 g	–
Soft soap	—	10 g
Distilled water added to	50 mL	50 mL

（2）Procedures.

a. Prescription I: Take sodium hydroxide, add 2 mL of water for stirring to dissolve. Stand for cooling to room temperature, add it to vegetable oil. Heat the mixture at 90 ℃ in a water bath, and stir constantly. When $50\% \sim 70\%$ of the solution converts into floccules, 1 mL of ethanol is added, and the mixture is cooled to room temperature under mild stirring. 20 min after standing, the mixture is heated in a water bath for 5 min. Then keep stirring until the viscosity of the mixture increases. Add 1 mL of ethanol and continue stirring until complete saponification (semi-solid). If the saponification is uncompleted, add extra 1 mL of ethanol and stir until complete saponification. Add cresol carefully while hot under stirring to make it dissolve completely. Finally stand for cooling and add distilled water to the whole volume of 50 mL.

b. Prescription II: Take 10 g of commercially available soft soap and cut into pieces, add 10 mL of cresol and stir to disperse uniformly. Add distilled water to the whole volume of 50 mL and stir completely.

c. Dilution test: Take 1 mL of cresol soap solutions of prescription I and II, respectively, and dilute with distilled water by $2 \sim 20$ times and then more than 200 times to observe the clarity of the solution.

[**Precautions**]

（1）Cresol and phenol possess similar physicochemical properties due to analogous structures. It is notable that the sterilization efficiency of cresol is much stronger than that of phenol. Cresol is irritant to skin at high concentrations, so be careful when handling. When the concentration of cresol in the air increases, it will be irritating to mucosa membranes.

（2）The solubility of cresol in water is low (1 : 50), and sodium soap produced by vegetable oil reacting with sodium hydroxide can solubilize cresol to prepare high concentration of cresol soap solution up to 50%. In the present experiment, the prepared cresolsoap solution is 20%.

(3) The degree of saponification is closely related to the quality of cresol soap solutions. The saponification can be accelerated by adding a small amount of ethanol. After the reaction accomplished, ethanol is evaporated by heating.

(4) The criteria judging for complete saponification: the product is semi-solid and has no obvious oil droplets or oil on the surface.

(5) Carefully add cresol to the newly formed soap in a hot state and rapidly stirred to dissolve (operating in a fume hood). Rapidly and carefully transfer it to a volumetric flask, preventing cresol from polluting air by volatilizing.

(6) The solution, prepared by cresol, soap and water, is a complex system which holds some characteristics of colloidal solutions. It is translucent and will not be opaque when diluted by water.

3. Preparation of Florida water

(1) Prescription:

Menthol	0. 2 g
Borneol	0. 2 g
Fragrance	1. 0 g
Pigment	q. s.
Anhydrous ethanol	70 mL
Distilled water added to	100 mL

(2) Procedures: Dissolve menthol and borneol with a small amount of anhydrous ethanol, add fragrance and pigment under stirring to dissolve. Then add the remaining ethanol under stirring to mix uniformly. Finally add distilled water to the whole volume of 100 mL, stand for one week at room temperature to age well and then pack into vials.

[**Precautions**]

(1) Menthol and borneol are easily soluble in anhydrous ethanol and slightly soluble in water. So they should be completely dissolved in ethanol before adding distilled water for dilution.

(2) Aging is to let menthol, borneol and ethanol stand for a period of time to fully react to form fatty acid esters with aroma, which makes the fragrance of the solution more concentrated and can mask or lighten the original pungent odor of ethanol, hence reducing the amount of flavor added.

4. Preparation of hand sanitizer

(1) Prescription:

Ethanol	65 mL
Carbomer 940	0. 4 g
Glycerol	5. 0 g
Fragrance	1. 0 g
Pigment	q. s.
Trolamine	q. s.
Distilled water added to	100 g

(2) Procedures:

a. Preparation of hand sanitizer: Take 25 mL of water, sprinkle carbomer 940 evenly on the surface of water to form a thin layer. After carbomer completely swollen (forming transparent gels), add ethanol and glycerol and stir to form transparent solution, and then add fragrance and appropriate amount of pigment under stirring. Finally, add trolamine (about 5～6 drops) to adjust pH to 7. 0, and then add distilled water to 100 g.

b. Evaluation of antibacterial effect: Take a sterile glass slide, drop 2 drops of sterile water on the slide. Take a sterile cotton bud pre-moistened with sterile water to scrape twice on the 5 fingers of a volunteer. Transfer thoroughly the bacteria collected on the cotton bud to water drop-let on the left side of the slide. The volunteer takes coin-sized hand sanitizer on the hands and repeatedly rubs to make the hand sanitizer evenly distributed on the hands. Pay special atten-tion, make the fingers and the palm fully contact with the hand sanitizer. One minute later, moisten the sterile cotton bud with sterilized water, scrape twice similarly on the five fingers of the homolateral hand of the volunteer. And then the bacteria collected on the cotton bud are transferred to water droplet on the right side of the slide. Fix and carry out Gram staining (De-tailed in Appendix ⅢA). Observe the change in the number and types of microorganisms be-fore and after using hand sanitizer under the microscope.

[Precautions]

Carbomer 940 swells slowly. Try to sprinkle it over a larger area of water to form a thin layer so as to accelerate the limited swelling process.

Ⅵ. Experiment results and discussion

(1) Describe the appearance of the compound iodine solution.

(2) Observe the appearance of prescriptions Ⅰ and Ⅱ of cresol soap solutions and the clarity after dilution.

Comparison of traits of cresol soap solution is detailed in Table 3 − 1.

Prescription	I	II
Table 3 – 1 Comparison of traits of cresol soap solution		
Cresol soap solution		
Diluted by 2 times		
Diluted by 20 times		
Diluted by more than 200 times		

（3）Antibacterial experiment. The number and types of bacteria on the hands before and after using the hand sanitizer is observed by an optical microscope for evaluating the antibacterial effect of the hand sanitizer.

VII. Questions

（1）Write down the saponification reaction equation in the cresol soap solutions experiment. What methods can be used to accelerate the rate of saponification reaction? Analyze the effect of ethanol in this experiment.

（2）What is the clinical significance that the cresol soap solution remains translucent when diluted by 2～20 times?

（3）What is the pharmacological effect of menthol and borneol in the formulation of Florida water? What should be paid more attention in this experiment?

实验二 混悬剂的制备及稳定剂的选择

一、实验目的

（1）掌握混悬剂的一般制备方法。
（2）掌握混悬剂的质量检查方法。
（3）熟悉混悬剂的稳定化原理和方法。

二、实验原理

混悬剂（suspensions）系指难溶性固体药物以微粒状态分散在液体介质中形成的非

均相分散体系。

混悬剂属于热力学不稳定体系，微粒的沉降是混悬剂物理不稳定性的主要表现。根据 Stokes 定律 $V = \dfrac{2r^2(\rho_1 - \rho_2)g}{9\eta}$，可通过将药物粉碎减小微粒半径（$r$），减小微粒与液体介质密度差（$\rho_1 - \rho_2$），以及加入助悬剂增加介质黏度（$\eta$）等方法降低混悬剂中微粒的沉降速度，提高混悬剂的稳定性。

混悬剂中微粒分散度大，具有较大的表面自由能，体系处于不稳定状态。由公式 $\Delta F = \delta_{SL} \cdot \Delta A$ 可知，微粒总表面自由能的变化（ΔF）取决于微粒固液界面张力（δ_{SL}）和微粒总表面积的变化（ΔA）。因此，①可通过在混悬剂中加入适当的表面活性剂降低 δ_{SL}，降低微粒表面自由能，使体系稳定；②加入适量的絮凝剂，使微粒 ζ 电位降至 $20 \sim 25$ mV，微粒发生轻微的絮凝，减小微粒的总表面积，从而降低表面自由能，形成疏松聚集体，易于分散；③可加入适量反絮凝剂，通过增大微粒的 ζ 电位，增大电荷斥力，从而减少微粒的聚集，使混悬剂流动性增加，易于倾倒，便于分装和使用。

混悬剂标签上应注明"用前摇匀"。为安全起见，剧毒药不宜制成混悬剂。混悬剂应具备以下要求：药物的化学性质稳定，在有效期内含量及有关物质符合要求；微粒沉降速度慢，沉降不应有结块现象，轻摇后应迅速均匀分散；粒子大小及液体的黏度均应符合要求，易于倾倒且分剂量准确；外用混悬剂应易于涂布，且不易被擦掉或流失。除装量、微生物限度等检查外，还应测定沉降体积比，要求沉降体积比不低于 0.90。

三、预习思考

（1）混悬剂的常用制备方法有哪些？
（2）混悬剂的质量要求有哪些？
（3）根据 Stokes 定律和 $\Delta F = \delta_{SL} \cdot \Delta A$ 公式，简述提高混悬剂稳定性的措施。

四、实验材料与仪器

1. 实验试剂与试药材料
炉甘石、氧化锌、硫酸钡、硫黄、樟脑、羟丙基甲基纤维素（HPMC E5）、三氯化铝、柠檬酸三钠、甘油、吐温 80。

2. 实验仪器
天平、研钵、容量瓶、量筒、烧杯、筛网（100 目）、25 mL 纳氏比色管、试管。

五、实验内容

1. 药物的亲水性/疏水性观察
取试管加少量蒸馏水，分别加入少许氧化锌、硫酸钡、硫黄、炉甘石、樟脑粉末，轻微振摇，观察粉末与水接触的现象。分辨哪些化合物亲水，哪些疏水。然后在试管中加入 1～2 滴吐温 80，轻微振摇，观察现象。

2. 不同处方炉甘石洗剂的制备及其稳定性比较

1）处方（表 3-2）：

表 3-2 炉甘石洗剂处方

处方号	1	2	3	4	5	6	7	8
炉甘石/g	3.0	3.0	3.0	3.0	3.0	3.0	3.0	3.0
氧化锌/g	1.5	1.5	1.5	1.5	1.5	1.5	1.5	1.5
甘油/g	1.5	1.5	1.5	1.5	1.5	1.5	1.5	1.5
HPMC E5/g	0.6	0.3					0.3	
三氯化铝/g	—	—	0.050	0.025	—	—	—	—
柠檬酸三钠/g	—	—	—	—	0.2	0.1	0.1	—
加蒸馏水至/mL	25	25	25	25	25	25	25	25

2）实验步骤：

（1）稳定剂溶液的配制：①将 HPMC E5 配成 6.0% 的水溶液，取用 5 或 10 mL。②将三氯化铝配成 0.5% 的水溶液，取用 5 或 10 mL。③将柠檬酸三钠配成 2.0% 的水溶液，取用 5 或 10 mL。

（2）称取过 100 目筛的炉甘石、氧化锌于研钵中，照表 3-2 加入稳定剂溶液或等积的蒸馏水研成糊状，加甘油研匀，少量多次转移至纳氏比色管中，加水至刻度，即得 1～8 号洗剂。其中 8 号未加稳定剂，作为对照。

3）质量检查：

（1）沉降体积比：将上述处方的洗剂用力振摇 1 min，在表 3-4 中记录沉降前的初始高度 H_0，随后静置 3 h，于不同时间点记录沉降高度 H，计算沉降体积比 $F = H/H_0$，并绘制洗剂的沉降曲线。

（2）放置 3 h 后，将比色管倒置翻转（±180°为 1 次），记录使管底沉降物分散完全的翻转次数。

注意事项

（1）8 个处方应注意平行操作，应选用粗细均匀的比色管，研磨的时间和力度应尽量保持一致。

（2）翻转比色管时避免产生泡沫。

3. 助悬剂用量对混悬剂稳定性的影响

在表 3-2 中处方 1 的基础上，分别改变 HPMC E5 用量为 0.15 g、0.30 g、0.60 g 和 0.90 g 并制备混悬剂，测定沉降体积比和翻转次数，比较助悬剂用量对混悬剂稳定性的影响。

4. 比较不同浓度三氯化铝的絮凝作用

配制 0.5% 的三氯化铝溶液，分别量取 0 mL、2.5 mL、5.0 mL、7.5 mL、10.0 mL，按表 3−2 的处方 3 制备混悬剂。混悬剂静置 3 h 后，测定其沉降体积比，并按公式 $\beta = F/F_\infty$ 计算絮凝度（β）。其中，F 为加有三氯化铝的混悬剂的沉降体积比，F_∞ 为未加三氯化铝混悬剂的沉降体积比。

六、实验结果与讨论

1. 药物亲水性与疏水性的观察

将药物亲水性与疏水性的观察结果填入表 3−3。

表 3−3　药物的亲水性/疏水性观察结果

药物	现象	亲水/疏水	加吐温 80 振摇后
氧化锌			
硫酸钡			
硫黄			
炉甘石			
樟脑			

2. 不同处方炉甘石洗剂稳定性比较

以沉降体积比 F 为纵坐标，沉降时间 t 为横坐标，分别绘制 8 个处方的沉降曲线，比较 8 个处方的稳定性（表 3−4）。

表 3−4　炉甘石洗剂沉降体积比和翻转次数

t/min	处方 1		处方 2		处方 3		处方 4		处方 5		处方 6		处方 7		处方 8	
	H/cm	F	H/cm	F	H/cm	F	H/cm	F	H/cm	F	H/cm	F	H/cm	F	H/cm	F
0																
10																
20																
30																
60																
120																
180																
翻转次数																

3. 助悬剂用量对混悬剂稳定性的影响

将实验结果填入表 3−5。

表3-5　含不同量助悬剂炉甘石洗剂的沉降体积比和翻转次数

序号	HPMC E5/g	H_0/cm	H/cm	F	翻转次数
1	0.15				
2	0.30				
3	0.60				
4	0.90				

4. 不同浓度三氯化铝溶液的絮凝作用

将实验结果填入表3-6。

表3-6　不同浓度三氯化铝对炉甘石洗剂絮凝度的影响

序号	三氯化铝体积/mL	H_0/cm	H/cm	F	β
1	0				
2	2.5				
3	5.5				
4	7.5				
5	10.0				

七、思考题

（1）絮凝剂与反絮凝剂的区别是什么？

（2）亲水性、疏水性、水溶性与水不溶性的区别与联系是什么？

（3）影响混悬剂稳定性的因素有哪些？查询几种市售混悬剂，找出处方中的稳定剂，说明其稳定机理。

Experiment 2　Preparation of Suspensions and Selection of Stabilizers

Ⅰ. Purpose

（1）To master conventional preparation methods of suspensions.

（2）To grasp quality inspections of suspensions.

（3）To be familiar with stabilization principles and various stabilization methods of suspensions.

Ⅱ. Principles

Suspensions is a heterogeneous dispersion system in which poorly soluble solid drugs disperse in liquid medium by particles.

Suspensions belongs to thermodynamic instability system, and the settling of particles is the main manifestation of the physical instability. According to Stokes' law $V = \dfrac{2r^2(\rho_1 - \rho_2)g}{9\eta}$, decreasing particle radius (r) by crushing drugs, eliminating the density difference between particles and liquid medium ($\rho_1 - \rho_2$), and increasing the medium viscosity (η) by adding suspending agents can reduce the sedimentation velocity (V) of particles in suspensions so as to improve the stability of suspensions.

The system is unstable, as particles in suspensions have high dispersion degree and huge surface free energy. According to the formula $\Delta F = \delta_{SL} \cdot \Delta A$, changes of total surface free energy of particles (ΔF) depends on the solid-liquid interfacial tension of particles (δ_{SL}) and changes of total surface area of particles (ΔA). Therefore, ① adding appropriate amount of surfactant to suspensions can decrease δ_{SL}, thus reduce the surface free energy of particles. ② Adding appropriate amount of flocculants can reduce the zeta potential of particles to a certain degree of $20 \sim 25$ mV, cause slightly flocculation, and reduce the total surface area of particles ΔA, thereby attenuating the surface free energy ΔF of the loose aggregation, and making it easy to be redispersed after vibrating. ③ Adding suitable amount of deflocculants can increase the zeta potential of particles and then increase the charge repulsion force, hence reduce the aggregation of particles, make it easy to pour out, subpackage and utilize.

Suspensions require labeling notice indicating "shake well prior to application". For security, highly toxic substance should not be prepared as suspensions. Requirements that suspensions should meet are shown as follows: drug is stable in liquid medium, the content and related substances meet the requirements within shelf life; the sedimentation velocity of particles is low and lump will not occur during sedimentation; suspensions can be quickly uniformly redistributed after gently shaking; particle size and liquid viscosity are appropriated for both easy pouring and accurate dosing; suspensions for external use should be easy-spreading and avoid being wiped off by accident. Besides filling and microbial limit, the ratio of sedimental volume should also be determined, and the ratio of sedimental volume should be not less than 0.90.

III. Preview

(1) What conventional methods are used to prepare suspensions?

(2) What quality inspections should suspensions meet?

(3) According to Stokes' law and formula $\Delta F = \delta_{SL} \cdot \Delta A$, briefly describe the methods on how to improve the stability of suspensions.

IV. Experiment materials and equipments

1. Reagents and experimental materials

Calamine, zinc oxide (ZnO), barium sulfate (BaSO$_4$), sulfur, camphor, hydroxy propyl methyl cellulose (HPMC E5), $AlCl_3$, sodium citrate, glycerol, Tween 80.

2. Experimental equipments

Balance, mortar, volumetric flask, measuring cylinder, beaker, 100-mesh sieve, Nessler tube (25 mL), test tube.

V. Experiment contents

1. Observe the hydrophilic/hydrophobic of drugs

Add ZnO, $BaSO_4$, sulfur, calamine and camphor respectively to the test tubes in which distilled water is pre-added. After gently shaking, observe the contact phenomena between drug powders and water. Identify drugs with hydrophilicity or hydrophobicity. Then add $1 \sim 2$ drops of Tween 80 to the test tubes with hydrophobic drugs, shake it slightly and observe the change.

2. Preparation and comparison the stability of calamine lotions with different stabilizers

1) Prescriptions (Table 3 −2):

Table 3 −2   Prescriptions of calamine lotion

Prescription Number	1	2	3	4	5	6	7	8
Calamine/g	3.0	3.0	3.0	3.0	3.0	3.0	3.0	3.0
ZnO/g	1.5	1.5	1.5	1.5	1.5	1.5	1.5	1.5
Glycerol/g	1.5	1.5	1.5	1.5	1.5	1.5	1.5	1.5
HPMC E5/g	0.6	0.3	—	—	—	—	0.3	—
$AlCl_3$/g	—	—	0.050	0.025	—	—	—	—
Sodiumcitrate/g	—	—	—	—	0.2	0.1	0.1	—
Add distilled water to/mL	25	25	25	25	25	25	25	25

2) Procedures:

(1) Preparation of stabilizer solution: ①Prepare 6.0% HPMC ES, take 5 or 10 mL as stabilizer. ②Prepare 0.5% $AlCl_3$, take 5 or 10 mL as stabilizer. ③Prepare 2.0% sodium citrate, take 5 or 10 mL as stabilizer.

(2) Pass calamine and ZnO through 100-mesh sieve respectively. According to Table 3 −2, put calamine and ZnO in mortar, and add stabilizer solution or equal volume of distilled water, mix by grinding to a smooth paste. And then add glycerol to grind uniformly, transfer them carefully to Nessler tube, add distilled water to full quantity to obtain calamine lotion 1 ∼ 8. Calamine lotion 8 is absent of stabilizer, which is served as control group.

3) Quality inspections:

(1) Ratio of sedimental volume: Shaking vigorously the above calamine lotion for 1 min and record the initial height (H_0), then stand for 3 h respectively, record sedimentation height (H) of fallout at different time points and fill in Table 3 −4, calculate the ratio of sedimental volume (F) according to formula $F = H/H_0$ and draw settlement curve of calamine lotions.

(2) After placing for 3 h, turn over the Nessler tube (±180° for once), and record the

turnover times until the sedimentation at the bottom of the tube completely dispersed.

[**Precautions**]

（1）The parallel operation of preparing suspensions is in strict demands. For example, select uniform Nessler tubes with the same internal diameter, the consistent grinding time and force.

（2）Avoid foam when flipping Nessler tubes.

3. The influence of the suspending agents dosage on the stability of suspensions

On the basis of prescription 1 in Table 3 – 2, change the dosage of HPMC E5 to 0. 15 g, 0. 30 g, 0. 60 g and 0. 90 g respectively to prepare suspensions. Measure the ratio of sedimental volume and turnover times to evaluate the influence of suspending agents dosage on the stability of suspensions.

4. Compare the flocculation effect of $AlCl_3$ at different concentrations

According to prescription 3 in Table 3 – 2, take 0 mL, 2. 5 mL, 5. 0 mL, 7. 5 mL, 10. 0 mL of 0. 5% $AlCl_3$ respectively to prepare the suspensions. After standing for 3 h, measure the ratio of sedimental volume, and calculate the flocculation value (β) according to formula $\beta = F/F_\infty$. Where F is the ratio of sedimental volume of suspensions with $AlCl_3$, and F_∞ is the ratio of sedimental volume of suspensions without $AlCl_3$.

VI. Experiment results and discussion

1. Hydrophilicity/hydrophobicity of drugs

Hydrophilicity/hydrophobicity of drugs is detailed in Table 3 – 3.

Table 3 – 3　Hydrophilicity/hydrophobicity of drugs

Drugs	Phenomenon	Hydrophilic/hydrophobic	Add Tween 80 and shake
ZnO			
$BaSO_4$			
Sulfur			
Calamine			
Camphor			

2. Stability of calamine lotions with different stabilizers

Take ratio of sedimental volume (F) as abscissa and sedimentation time as ordinates, draw settlement curve of 8 prescriptions respectively and compare the stability of various prescriptions (Table 3 – 4).

Table 3 -4   Ratio of sedimental volume and turnover times of calamine lotions

t/min	Prescription 1		Prescription 2		Prescription 3		Prescription 4		Prescription 5		Prescription 6		Prescription 7		Prescription 8	
	H/cm	F	H/cm	F	H/cm	F	H/cm	F	H/cm	F	H/cm	F	H/cm	F	H/cm	F
0																
10																
20																
30																
60																
120																
180																
Turnover times																

3. The effect of suspending agents dosage on the stability of suspensions

The effect of suspending agents dosage on the stability of suspensions is detailed in Table 3 -5.

Table 3 -5   Ratio of sedimental volume and turnover times of calamine lotions with various dosage of suspending agents

Number	HPMC E5/g	H_0/cm	H/cm	F	Turnover times
1	0.15				
2	0.30				
3	0.60				
4	0.90				

4. Flocculation effect of $AlCl_3$ at different concentrations

Flocculation effect of $AlCl_3$ at different concentrations is detailed in Table 3 -6.

Table 3 -6   Flocculation values of calamine lotion at different $AlCl_3$ concentrations

Number	Volume of $AlCl_3$/mL	H_0/cm	H/cm	F	β
1	0				
2	2.5				
3	5.0				
4	7.5				
5	10.0				

VII. Questions

(1) Please describe the differences between flocculants and defloculants.

(2) Please describe the differences between hydrophilic and hydrophobic, between water-soluble and water-insoluble.

(3) What factors affect the stability of suspensions? Search for several commercially available suspensions and find out the stabilizers in the prescriptions, and explain the stabilization mechanism.

实验三 乳剂的制备与评价

一、实验目的

（1）掌握乳剂的一般制备方法。

（2）掌握乳剂的类型及其关键决定因素。

（3）熟悉乳剂的处方组成和乳化方法对乳滴大小的影响。

（4）熟悉乳剂的质量检查方法。

（5）了解乳化油相所需乳化剂的亲水亲油平衡（hydrophilic lipophilic balance，*HLB*）值的确定方法。

二、实验原理

乳剂（emulsions）系指互不相溶的两种液体混合，其中一种液体以小液滴状均匀分散于另一种液体中而形成的非均相液体制剂，属于热力学不稳定体系。

乳剂由水相（W）、油相（O）和乳化剂组成。根据结构的不同，乳剂可分为简单乳和复合乳；根据分散相性质的不同，可分为水包油（O/W）型和油包水（W/O）型；根据液滴的大小，可分为普通乳、亚微乳和微乳。乳剂的类型主要取决于乳化剂的种类、性质和两相体积比，通常采用稀释法或染色法进行鉴别。

乳剂中的液滴分散度高，总表面积大，因此有较高的表面自由能。根据 $\Delta F = \delta_{LL} \times \Delta A$，液滴有自动合并成更大液滴、减少总表面积、降低体系自由能的趋势。因此，在机械力作用下，将机械能转变为表面能，同时加入乳化剂显著降低油-水界面张力，并在乳滴周围形成牢固的乳化膜，防止液滴合并，能制备优质的乳剂。常用的乳化剂有：①表面活性剂类乳化剂，如脱水山梨醇脂肪酸酯（司盘）类和聚氧乙烯脱水山梨醇脂肪酸酯（吐温）类；②亲水高分子乳化剂，如阿拉伯胶和西黄蓍胶；③固体微粒乳化剂，如二氧化硅和氢氧化钙；④辅助乳化剂，如长链脂肪醇。

表面活性剂的亲水性或亲脂性是由变量 *HLB* 值来衡量的。在乳剂制备时，应选择适宜 *HLB* 值的乳化剂。单一乳化剂难以符合精准 *HLB* 值的要求，通常使用复合乳化剂，其相比于单一乳化剂乳化效果更好。非离子表面活性剂的 *HLB* 值具有加和性，2 种或以上表面活性剂混合后的 *HLB* 值可按式（3-3-1）计算：

$$HLB_{AB} = \frac{HLB_A \times W_A + HLB_B \times W_B}{W_A + W_B} \qquad (3-3-1)$$

式中，W_A 和 W_B 分别表示表面活性剂 A 和 B 的质量，HLB_A 和 HLB_B 则分别是 A 和 B 各自的 HLB 值，HLB_{AB} 为混合后的表面活性剂的 HLB 值。

乳化油相所需乳化剂的最适 HLB 值也可通过实验筛选，即通过配制不同 HLB 值的复合乳化剂，制得系列乳剂并比较它们的稳定性。能形成理化性质适宜、稳定性良好的乳液的复合乳化剂，其 HLB 值称为乳化剂的最适 HLB 值。

乳剂的制备方法有干胶法、湿胶法、新生皂法和机械法等。制备工艺流程见图 3-1～图 3-4。

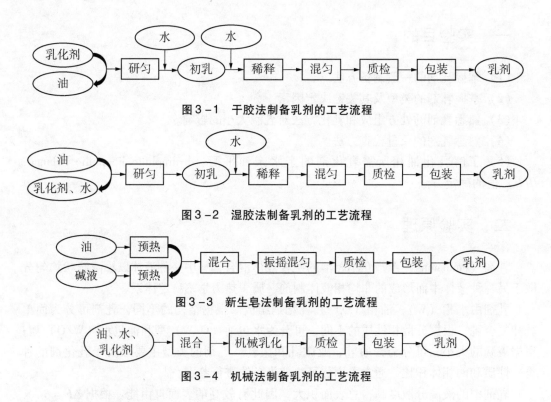

图 3-1　干胶法制备乳剂的工艺流程

图 3-2　湿胶法制备乳剂的工艺流程

图 3-3　新生皂法制备乳剂的工艺流程

图 3-4　机械法制备乳剂的工艺流程

三、预习思考

（1）根据结构、分散相组成以及液滴大小，可以将乳剂可为哪几类？

（2）为什么乳化剂对于乳剂的形成是不可或缺的？乳剂形成的机制是什么？

（3）乳化剂可分为哪几类？请简述其特点和适用范围。

（4）请分析使用高速分散均质机的注意事项。

四、实验材料与仪器

1. 实验试剂与试药

阿拉伯胶、西黄蓍胶、花生油、吐温 80、司盘 80、氢氧化钙、亚甲蓝染料、苏丹 - Ⅳ染料、蒸馏水。

2. 实验仪器

恒温水浴锅、高速分散均质机、离心机、天平、紫外 – 可见分光光度计、显微镜、研钵、烧杯、量筒、具塞试管、玻璃棒。

五、实验内容

（一）干胶法制备乳剂

1. 处方

花生油	11.8 g
阿拉伯胶	3.1 g
西黄蓍胶	0.4 g
蒸馏水加至	50 mL

2. 实验步骤

（1）称取处方量花生油、阿拉伯胶及西黄蓍胶加入研钵中研磨均匀，一次性加入蒸馏水 10 mL，快速用力向同一方向研磨。听到轻微"噼啪"声，提示初乳形成，得外观为白色或类白色黏稠状液体。

（2）用蒸馏水将初乳分次洗涤转移至量筒，加水至 50 mL，混匀，即得。

注意事项

（1）制备初乳的研钵应保持干燥，研钵和研棒表面粗糙有利于初乳形成。

（2）初乳的形成是干胶法制备乳剂的关键，研磨时宜快速且用力均匀。

（3）制备初乳时，水的比例过低或加水速度过慢均易形成 W/O 型初乳，此时加水稀释也难以转变为 O/W 型；若水的比例过高，会导致水相黏度低，对油的分散能力低，制得的初乳大多不稳定或容易破裂。

（二）比较手工法与机械法制备乳剂

1. 处方

花生油	10.9 g
吐温 80	5.4 g
蒸馏水加至	100 mL

2. 实验步骤

（1）手工法：取以上处方量的一半进行操作，在烧杯中加入吐温 80 和花生油，搅拌混匀，加入 4 mL 水搅拌，制备得白色黏稠状初乳，用蒸馏水稀释至 50 mL，即得。

（2）机械法：取处方量的花生油和吐温 80，加入 80 mL 水，调节高速分散均质机转速为 1 200～1 800 r/min，均质化 1 min，停机 30 s，再均质化 1 min，用蒸馏水稀释至 100 mL，即得。

注意事项

（1）机械法制备乳剂无须考虑组分的加入顺序，而是借助强大的机械力将机械能转变成表面能形成乳剂。

（2）机械法制备乳剂时，高速分散均质机的分散头要完全浸没在液体中，分散头底端需离容器底部至少 0.5 cm。

（三）新生皂法制备乳剂

1. 处方

氢氧化钙溶液	15 mL
花生油	15 mL

2. 实验步骤

（1）取新鲜配制的饱和氢氧化钙溶液于具塞试管中，置 80 ℃水浴中预热 15 min。

（2）取花生油置于 80 ℃水浴中预热 15 min。

（3）将花生油趁热倒入饱和氢氧化钙溶液中，加塞，用力振摇 5 min（中途需放气）至乳剂生成，临床上称为石灰搽剂。

（四）花生油乳化所需乳化剂 *HLB* 值的测定

1. 处方

花生油	10 mL
混合乳化剂	1 g
蒸馏水加至	20 mL

2. 实验步骤

（1）称取一定量司盘 80、吐温 80 配成六种混合乳化剂，使其 *HLB* 值为 4.3～14.0（计算司盘 80 和吐温 80 的用量，填于表 3-7 中）。

（2）取 6 支具塞刻度试管，加入花生油 10 mL，再分别加入上述不同 *HLB* 值的混合乳化剂各 1 g，然后加蒸馏水至 20 mL，加塞，用力振摇 2 min，形成乳剂，记录乳剂初始高度 H_0。放置 5 min、10 min、30 min 和 60 min 后，分别观察各乳剂分层的程度，记录乳剂的液体最终高度 H，计算沉降体积比（F）：$F = H/H_0$。

表3-7　复合乳化剂组成

编号	1	2	3	4	5	6
混合乳化剂 HLB 值	4.3	6.0	8.0	10.0	12.0	14.0
司盘80/g						
吐温80/g						

注：司盘80的 HLB 值为4.3，吐温80的 HLB 值为15.0。

注意事项

振摇6支具塞试管时，振摇强度应保持一致，同时准确控制振摇时间。

六、实验结果与讨论

1. 乳剂类型的鉴别

（1）稀释法：取乳剂少许，加水稀释。若能稀释成稳定的乳剂，则为 O/W 型，否则为 W/O 型。

（2）染色法：取乳剂少量涂于载玻片上，滴加油溶性染料苏丹-Ⅳ（1 mg/mL）以及水溶性染料亚甲基蓝（1 mg/mL）分别染色，用玻棒搅匀，加盖玻片。在显微镜下观察。能被苏丹-Ⅳ均匀分散的乳剂为 W/O 型乳剂，被亚甲基蓝均匀分散的则为 O/W型。将整体实验结果，填入表3-8中。

表3-8　乳剂类型的鉴别

乳化剂	阿拉伯胶	吐温80	新生皂
颜色			
稀释法			
染色			
滤纸上的扩散系数			
乳剂类型			

2. 乳剂粒径的测定

用配有测微尺的显微镜观察各个处方乳剂的最大粒径和最多粒径（详见附录ⅢB），并将结果填入表3-9中。

表3-9　乳剂粒径观察

实验处方号	最大粒径/μm	最多粒径/μm
处方1（干胶法）		
处方2（吐温80手工法）		
处方3（吐温80机械法）		
处方4（新生皂法）		

3. 稳定常数的测定

分别取乳剂 4 mL 置于 10 mL 离心管中，3 000 r/min 离心 10 min。自离心管底部吸取 50 μL 于 25 mL 容量瓶，加水稀释至刻度，摇匀。以蒸馏水为空白，测定 550 nm 处的吸收度，记为 A_t。同法吸取新鲜制备的、未离心乳剂样品 50 μL，稀释后测定 550 nm 处的吸收度，记为 A_0。根据式（3 – 3 – 2）计算乳剂的稳定参数 K_E：

$$K_E = \frac{A_0 - A_t}{A_0} \times 100\% \qquad (3 - 3 - 2)$$

式中，K_E 绝对值越小，乳剂越稳定。

将测得的结果填入表 3 – 10。

表 3 –10　不同方法制备乳剂的稳定常数

吸收度（$\lambda_{550\,nm}$）	手工法	机械法
离心前（A_0）		
离心后（A_t）		
稳定性参数（K_E）		

4. 花生油所需 *HLB* 值的测定

6 支具塞刻度试管加入花生油和乳化剂振摇后静置，观察并记录不同时间点各乳剂分层前后的高度（H 和 H_0），计算沉降体积比 F（表 3 – 11）。

表 3 –11　花生油所需 *HLB* 值测定结果

t/min	乳化剂 *HLB* 值											
	4.3		6.0		8.0		10.0		12.0		14.0	
	H/cm	F/%	H/cm	F/%	H/cm	F/%	H/cm	F/%	H/cm	F/%	H/cm	F/%
0												
5												
10												
30												
60												

乳化花生油所需 *HLB* 值为_____，所制得的乳剂的类型为_____

七、思考题

（1）影响乳剂类型的主要因素有哪些？

（2）简述干胶法与湿胶法制备初乳的操作要点。

（3）筛选乳化油相所需乳化剂的 *HLB* 值有何意义？

Experiment 3 Preparation and Quality Inspections of Emulsions

I. Purpose

(1) To master the conventional preparation methods of emulsions.

(2) To master the classification of emulsions and their key determinants.

(3) To be familiar with the effects of formulation components and emulsification methods on the droplet sizes.

(4) To be familiar with quality inspections of emulsions.

(5) To understand the method to determine hydrophile lipophile balance (HLB) values of emulsifiers required for the emulsification of oils.

II. Principles

Emulsions are two-phase, thermodynamically unstable systems, made of two immiscible liquids in which one liquid is dispersed throughout another in the form of small droplets.

Emulsions usually consist of aqueous phase (W), oil phase (O) and emulsifiers, which are divided into simple emulsions and compound emulsions by their structure. In addition, according to the features of the dispersed phase, emulsions are divided into oil-in-water (O/W) type and water-in-oil (W/O) type. While base on the droplet sizes, they are divided into ordinary emulsions, submicron emulsions and microemulsions. The types of emulsions mostly depend on the types of emulsifiers and the phase volume fraction, which can be easily distinguished by dilution methods or differential staining.

The droplets possess high dispersion degree, huge total surface area and therefore high surface free energy. According to the formula $\Delta F = \delta_{LL} \times \Delta A$, droplets prone to merge automatically to form larger droplets, resulting in decreased total surface area and surface free energy. Hence the formation of emulsions is a process that converting mechanical energy into surface energy in the presence of mechanical force. Meanwhile, emulsifiers are required to significantly reduce the oil-water interfacial tension and form emulsifying layer around the scattered droplets to prevent coalescence. Commonly used emulsifiers include: ① surfactants such as sorbitan fatty acid ester derivatives (Span) and polyoxyethylene sorbitol fatty acid ester derivatives (Tween); ② hydrophilic polymers such as gum arabic and tragacanth; ③ solid particles such as silica and calcium hydroxide; ④ co-emulsifiers such as long-chain fatty alcohol.

The hydrophilicity or lipophilicity of surfactants is measured in terms of variable hydrophilic lipophilic balance (*HLB*) value. Emulsions are usually stable when emulsifiers with suitable *HLB* value are used. The single emulsifier is usually difficult to meet the requirements for *HLB* value, and compound emulsifiers therefore are better based on the additive property of their *HLB* values. The *HLB* value of nonionic surfactants is additive, so the formula (3 – 3 – 1) can be used to calculate the *HLB* value of two or more surfactants after mixing.

$$HLB_{AB} = \frac{HLB_A \times W_A + HLB_B \times W_B}{W_A + W_B} \qquad (3-3-1)$$

In the formula, W_A and W_B represent the weight of surfactant A and B respectively, HLB_A and HLB_B are the *HLB* values of A and B respectively, HLB_{AB} is the mixed surfactant *HLB* value.

In general, the optimum *HLB* value of emulsifiers required for emulsifying oil can also be selected by experiments; that is, preparing a series of emulsions by compound emulsifiers with different *HLB* values and comparing their stability. The *HLB* value of compound emulsifiers that form stable emulsions possessing suitable physicochemical properties is called the appropriate *HLB* value of emulsifiers for this oil.

The preparation methods of emulsions include dry gum method, wet gum method, nascent soap method, mechanical method and so on. The preparation processes are detailed in Figure 3-1 to Figure 3-4.

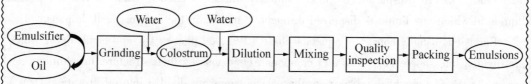

Figure 3-1　Preparation of emulsions by dry gum method

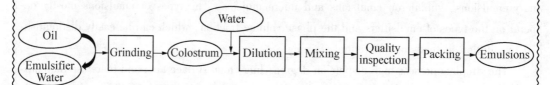

Figure 3-2　Preparation of emulsions by wet gum method

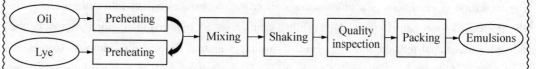

Figure 3-3　Preparation of emulsions by nascent soap method

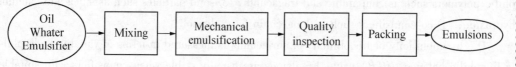

Figure 3-4　Preparation of emulsions by mechanical method

Ⅲ. Preview

(1) Which types are emulsions classified according to the structure, dispersed phase composition, and droplet sizes?

(2) Why are emulsifiers indispensable for the emulsions formation? What is the mechanisms of emulsion formation?

(3) How many types can emulsifiers be divided into? Please describe their characteristics and the extent of application in brief.

(4) Please describe the precautions when use high speed dispersion homogenizer.

Ⅳ. Experiment materials and equipments

1. Reagents and experimental materials

Gum arabic, tragacanth, peanut oil, Tween 80, Span 80, calcium hydroxide, methylene blue, Sudan-Ⅳ, distilled water.

2. Experimental equipments

Constant temperature water bath, high speed dispersion homogenizer, centrifuge, balance, UV-visible spectrophotometer, microscope, mortar, beaker, volumetric cylinder, test tube with glass stopper, glass rod.

Ⅴ. Experiment contents

1. Preparation of emulsions by dry gum method

1) Prescription:

Peanut oil	11.8 g
Gum arabic	3.1 g
Tragacanth	0.4 g
Distilled water added to	50 mL

2) Procedures:

(1) Add peanut oil, gum arabic and tragacanth into a mortar and grind to promote uniformity, and then add distilled water 10 mL. Grind quickly, vigorously in the same direction until a slight sputter sound occurs, indicating emulsions are formed as the primary emulsions characterized by white or off-white viscous liquids.

(2) Transfer the primary emulsions to the volumetric cylinder, then wash and add with distilled water to 50 mL.

[**Precautions**]

(1) Dry and scobinate mortars are recommended to prepare primary emulsions.

(2) The formation of primary emulsions is critical for preparing emulsions by dry gum method. Grinding quickly and vigorously would be better.

(3) Water-in-oil primary emulsions would be formed when the proportion of water is excessive low or adding velocity is excessive slow, even it is hard to convert to oil-in-water emulsions after dilution. However, high proportion of water will result in aqueous phase with low viscosity, which is hard to disperse oil, and the primary emulsions obtained is unstable and emulsions rupture easily occurs.

2. Comparison of manual and mechanical methods in preparing emulsions

1) Prescription:

Peanut oil	10.9 g
Tween 80	5.4 g
Distilled water added to	100 mL

2) Procedures:

(1) Manual method: Take half of the above prescription for preparation. Put Tween 80 and peanut oil to a beaker, then add 4 mL water and stir. Finally, the obtained white viscous primary emulsions are diluted by distilled water to 50 mL.

(2) Mechanical method: Put peanut oil, Tween 80 and 80 mL water to a beaker under the high-speed dispersion homogenizer. Adjust the speed to 1 200 ~ 1 800 r/min and homogenize for 1 min, where stop for 30 s and homogenize for the next 1 min. Finally, the obtained primary emulsions are diluted by distilled water to 100 mL.

[**Precautions**]

(1) Preparing emulsions by mechanical method utilizes powerful mechanical force to convert mechanical energy to surface energy, thus it is unnecessary to consider the adding order of different components.

(2) When preparing emulsions by mechanical method, the dispersing head of the high-speed dispersing homogenizer should be completely immersed in the mixed liquids, where the head should be at least 0.5 cm away from the bottom of the container.

3. Preparation of emulsions by nascent soap method

1) Prescription:

Calcium hydroxide solution	15 mL
Peanut oil	15 mL

2）Procedures：

（1）Put freshly prepared saturated calcium hydroxide solution in a test tube with glass stopper, preheat the tube at 80 ℃ in water bath for 15 min.

（2）Preheat peanut oil at 80 ℃ in water bath for 15 min.

3）Pour peanut oil into the saturated calcium hydroxide solution while it's hot, add stopper and shake vigorously for 5 min（outgassing constantly）to prepare emulsions, which is called lime liniments clinically.

4. Determination of *HLB* value for emulsifying peanut oil

1）Prescription：

Peanut oil	10 mL
Mixed emulsifiers	1 g
Distilled water added to	20 mL

2）Procedures：

（1）Weigh a certain amount of Span 80 and Tween 80, and mix them to prepare six compound emulsifiers with *HLB* values from 4.3 to 14.0（Calculate the amount of Span 80 and Tween 80 used, and fill the result in Table 3 – 7）.

（2）Add 10 mL of peanut oil and 1 g compound emulsifiers mentioned above to 6 test tubes with stoppers. Add distilled water to 20 mL, add stopper and shake vigorously for 2 min to form emulsions, and record height H_0 at the beginning. Stand for 5 min, 10 min, 30 min and 60 min, observe the delamination of each emulsion and record the final height H. Calculate the ratio of sedimental volume（F）, $F = H/H_0$.

Table 3 –7　Composition of compound emulsifiers

Number	1	2	3	4	5	6
HLB value	4.3	6.0	8.0	10.0	12.0	14.0
Span 80/g						
Tween 80/g						

Notice：*HLB* value of Span 80 is 4.3；*HLB* value of Tween 80 is 15.0.

[**Precautions**]

The shaking strength should be consistent and the shaking time should be controlled accurately.

VI. Experiment results and discussion

1. Identification of the types of emulsions

(1) Tube dilution method. the emulsions which can be diluted with water and stable retentively are O/W emulsions, otherwise are W/O emulsions.

(2) Staining method. Put a blob of emulsions on the glass slide, add oil-soluble dye Sudan-Ⅳ solution (1 mg/mL) and the water-soluble dye methylene blue solution (1 mg/mL) respectively. Mix emulsions by a glass rod, then cover the slide. Observing under the microscope, emulsions that can be dispersed in Sudan-Ⅳ are W/O emulsions while dispersed in methylene blue are O/W emulsions. Fill the results in Table 3 – 8.

Table 3 –8　Identification of the types of emulsions

Emulsifiers	Gum arabic	Tween 80	Nascent soap
Color			
Tube dilution method			
Staining method			
Diffusion velocity on filter paper			
Types of emulsions			

2. Measurement of droplet sizes of emulsions

The maximum of droplet sizes and the widest distribution of droplet sizes of each emulsion are observed under a microscope equipped with a micrometer (See Appendix ⅢB for detail). Fill the results in Table 3 –9.

Table 3 –9　Droplet sizes of emulsions

Prescription	The maximum size/μm	The widest distribution of droplet sizes/μm
Dry gum method		
Tween 80 by manual method		
Tween 80 by mechanical method		
Nascent soap method		

3. Determining the stability constant of emulsions

Put 4 mL of emulsions into a 10 mL centrifuge tube and centrifuge at 3 000 r/min for 10 min. Pipette 50 μL emulsions from the bottom of the tube into a 25 mL volumetric flask, add distilled water to the scale and shake well. Determine the absorbance of emulsions at 550 nm with distilled water as blank control and denoted as A_t. Similarly, dilute 50 μL of freshly prepared, uncentrifuged emulsions with distilled water to 25 mL, determine the absorbance at 550 nm and denoted as A_0. Use the formula (3 –3 –2) to calculate the stability parameter K_E of the emulsions:

$$K_E = \frac{A_0 - A_t}{A_0} \times 100\% \tag{3 – 3 – 2}$$

The smaller K_E is, the more stable emulsions are.

Fill the results in Table 3 – 10.

Table 3 – 10　Stability constants of emulsions prepared by different methods

Absorbance ($\lambda_{550\ nm}$)	Manual method	Mechanical method
Before centrifugation (A_0)		
After centrifugation (A_t)		
Stability constant (K_E)		

4. Determination of *HLB* value required for emulsifying peanut oil

After standing for different time, record the height (H and H_0) of emulsions, and calculate the ratio of sedimental volume F. Fill the results in Table 3 – 11.

Table 3 – 11　*HLB* value required for emulsifying peanut oil

t/min	*HLB* value of emulsifiers											
	4. 3		6. 0		8. 0		10. 0		12. 0		14. 0	
	H/cm	F/%	H/cm	F/%	H/cm	F/%	H/cm	F/%	H/cm	F/%	H/cm	F/%
0												
5												
10												
30												
60												

The required *HLB* value for peanut oil is _____, and the type of emulsions is _____

VII. Questions

(1) What are the decisive factors for the formation of O/W or W/O emulsions?

(2) Describe the critical procedures of preparing primary emulsions by dry gum method and wet gum method.

(3) What is the significance of screening the *HLB* value of the emulsifiers required for emulsifying oil?

实验四　维生素 C 注射液的制备及处方工艺考察

一、实验目的

（1）掌握注射剂的生产工艺和操作要点。

（2）掌握注射剂的质量检查项目和方法。

（3）掌握影响维生素 C 注射液稳定性的因素及稳定化方法。

（4）熟悉考察注射剂稳定性的一般试验方法。

二、实验原理

注射剂（injections）又称针剂，系指由原料药物与适宜的辅料制成的供注入体内的无菌制剂。

注射剂分为注射液、注射用无菌粉末及注射用浓缩液等。注射液系指由药物与适宜的辅料制成的供注入体内的无菌液体制剂，包括溶液型注射液、混悬型注射液、乳剂型注射液。根据给药途径的不同，可分为静脉注射、肌内注射、鞘内注射、椎管内注射、皮下注射和皮内注射等。注射剂直接注入人体内部，具有吸收快、作用迅速的特点。为保证用药的安全性和有效性，必须对注射液生产和质量进行严格控制。

常见的溶液型注射剂的制备工艺如图 3-5 所示。

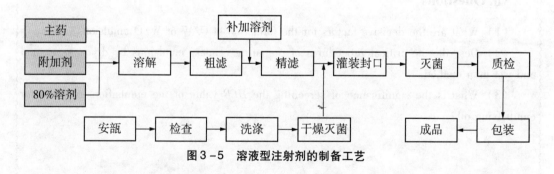

图 3-5　溶液型注射剂的制备工艺

注射剂质量检查包括无菌检查、细菌内毒素或热原检查、可见异物检查、pH 测定、装量、渗透压（大容量注射剂）和含量测定等，在有效期内均应符合要求。注射液的 pH 应接近体液，范围一般控制在 4～9。具体注射剂品种的 pH 的确定主要依据以下三个方面：满足临床需要；满足制剂制备、贮藏和使用时的稳定性要求；具有人体生理可承受性。凡大量静脉注射或滴注的输液，应调节其渗透压与血浆渗透压相等或接近。在水溶液中不稳定的药物常制成注射用灭菌粉末，即无菌冻干粉针或无菌粉末分装粉针，以保证注射剂在贮存期内稳定、安全、有效。

为了达到上述质量要求，在注射剂制备过程中，除了生产操作区需符合药品生产质量管理规范（Good Manufacturing Practices，GMP）要求和操作者严格遵守 GMP 规程，药物、附加剂及溶剂等均需符合注射用质量标准，其处方必须采用法定处方，制备方法必须严格遵守拟定的产品生产工艺规程，不得随意更改。

维生素 C 又被称为抗坏血酸，化学结构式如图 3 - 6 所示。结构中含有两个烯醇基，很容易被氧化，其氧化在有氧和无氧条件下均可进行。影响维生素 C 溶液稳定性的因素有很多，如氧气、pH、金属离子、温度、光线、水分及湿度等。维生素 C 不稳定性主要表现为放置过程中色泽变黄及含量下降。此外，维生素 C 分子中有烯二醇式结构，显强酸性，注射时刺激性大。因此，维生素 C 注射液的制备需考虑维生素 C 的稳定性及人体的耐受性。

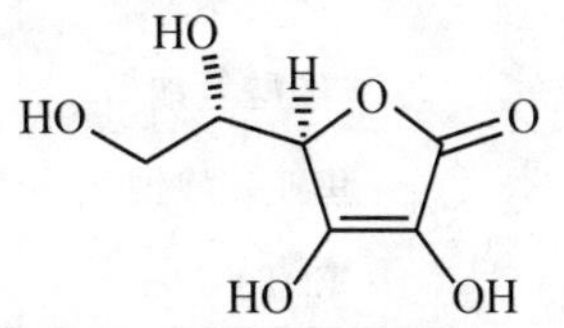

图 3 - 6　维生素 C 结构式

三、预习思考

（1）根据维生素 C 的结构特点，简述其理化性质。
（2）影响维生素 C 溶液稳定性的因素有哪些，如何提高稳定性？请填写至表 3 - 12。
（3）常用的抗氧化剂、pH 调节剂和金属螯合剂有哪些？
（4）如何考察维生素 C 注射液的稳定性？

表 3 - 12　影响维生素 C 溶液稳定性的因素以及相应的解决方法

	影响因素	解决措施
1		
2		
3		
4		
5		

四、实验材料与仪器

1. 实验试剂与试药

维生素 C、碳酸氢钠（$NaHCO_3$）、焦亚硫酸钠（$Na_2S_2O_5$）、硫酸铜（$CuSO_4$）、乙二胺四乙酸二钠（EDTA-2Na，别名依地酸二钠）、亚甲蓝、注射用水。

2. 实验仪器

紫外 - 可见分光光度计、pH 计、水浴锅、电炉、安瓿熔封机、容量瓶、烧杯、澄明度检测仪。

五、实验内容

1. 5%维生素 C 注射液的制备

1）处方：

维生素 C	2.50 g
碳酸氢钠	适量
焦亚硫酸钠	0.120 g
EDTA-2Na	0.125 g
注射用水加至	50 mL

2）实验步骤：

（1）空安瓿的处理。将安瓿中灌入常用水甩洗 2 次，再灌入蒸馏水甩洗 2 次。如果安瓿清洁度差，可用 0.1%盐酸灌入安瓿，100 ℃、30 min 热处理后再洗涤。洗净的安瓿倒放在烧杯内，120～140 ℃烘干备用。

（2）药液的配制。取注射用水加热煮沸，放冷至室温。取约 40 mL 放冷的注射用水，依次加入 EDTA-2Na 和维生素 C，搅拌溶解，加入焦亚硫酸钠。待溶解完全后，分次缓慢加入碳酸氢钠并不断搅拌至无气泡产生，使药液 pH 为 5.8～6.2，最后加注射用水稀释至 50 mL。

（3）灌封。用注射器吸取注射液，经 0.22 μm 微孔滤膜过滤，灌注 2.15 mL 于安瓿中，在瓶内液面下通入 CO_2 饱和后，立即熔封。安瓿熔封机的使用说明详见附录 IB。

（4）灭菌与检漏。注射液 100 ℃流通蒸汽灭菌 15 min。灭菌结束将安瓿放入有色水（如 1%的亚甲蓝溶液）中检漏，挑出变色的安瓿。

（5）注射液的质量检查。

A. 装量。取供试品 5 支，开启时注意避免损失，将内容物分别用相应体积的干燥注射器及注射针头抽尽，然后缓慢连续地注入经标化的量入式量筒内（量筒的大小应使待测体积至少占其额定体积的 40%，不排尽针头中的液体），在室温下检视。每支的装量均不得少于其标示量。

B. 可见异物检查。取供试品 20 支，除去容器标签，擦净容器外壁，置于澄明度检测仪（使用说明详见附录 IC）的遮光板边缘处。手持容器颈部，轻轻旋转和翻转容器（应避免产生气泡），使药液中可能存在的可见异物悬浮。分别在黑色和白色背景下目视检查，重复观察，总检查时限为 20 s，每次检查可手持 2 支。当有气泡产生影响观察时，需静置至气泡消失后重新检查。检查时被观察供试品处的光照度应为 1 000～1 500 lx。

C. 结果判定。供试品中不得检出金属屑、玻璃屑、长度超过 2 mm 的纤维、最大粒径超过 2 mm 的块状物和静置一定时间后轻轻旋转时肉眼可见的烟雾状微粒沉积物、无法计数的微粒群或摇不散的沉淀，以及在规定时间内较难计数的蛋白质絮状物等明显可见异物。如检出点状物、2 mm 以下的短纤维和块状物等微细可见异物，应符合表3-13中的规定。

表 3 – 13 非生物制品注射液的结果判定

类别		微细可见异物限度	
		初试 20 支	初、复试 40 支
注射液	静脉用	若 1 支检出，复试；若 2 支或以上检出，不符合规定	超过 1 支检出，不符合规定
	非静脉用	若 1～2 支检出，复试；如 2 支以上检出，不符合规定	超过 2 支检出，不符合规定

2. 对维生素 C 注射液稳定性的影响

取注射用水 400 mL 煮沸，放冷至室温，备用。取 15 g 维生素 C，加放冷至室温的注射用水溶解并稀释至 300 mL，制成 5% 的维生素 C 溶液，备用。取适量在 420 nm 处测定吸光度，记为 A_0。

（1）pH 的影响。

分别取 5% 的维生素 C 溶液 50 mL、200 mL、50 mL，用 $NaHCO_3$ 分别调节药液 pH 至 4.0 mL、6.0 mL 和 7.0 mL。用注射器吸取注射液 2 mL 灌装于 2 mL 安瓿中，立即熔封。不同 pH 的溶液各制备 20 支。

（2）空气中氧的影响。

称取 2.5 g 维生素 C 溶于未煮沸的 50 mL 水中，加 $NaHCO_3$ 粉末调节 pH 至 6.0，取 2 mL 灌入安瓿中，共灌封 20 支。另取步骤（1）中制备的 pH 为 6.0 的 5% 维生素 C 溶液 100 mL，微孔滤膜过滤后分成 2 份：①取 1 mL 灌入安瓿中，灌封 20 支；②取 2 mL 灌入安瓿中后，在瓶内液面下通入 CO_2（约 5 s），立即熔封，灌封 20 支。

（3）抗氧剂的影响。

取步骤（1）中制备的 pH 为 6.0 的维生素 C 溶液 50 mL，加入 0.12 g $Na_2S_2O_5$。待溶解完全后用微孔滤膜过滤，取 1 mL 滤液灌入安瓿中，灌封 20 支（图 3 – 7）。

（4）金属离子的影响。

取 5 g 维生素 C，加放冷至室温的注射用水溶解并稀释至 50 mL，用 $NaHCO_3$ 粉末调节 pH 至 6.0，制成 10% 维生素 C 溶液，分成 2 份，每份 25 mL。一份依次加入 5% EDTA-2Na 溶液 2.5 mL 和 0.1 mmol/L $CuSO_4$ 溶液 12.5 mL，加水定容至 50 mL；另一份中仅加入 0.1 mmol/L $CuSO_4$ 溶液 12.5 mL，加水定容至 50 mL（图 3 – 8）。分别取上述两种溶液 2 mL 灌装于 2 mL 安瓿中，各灌封 20 支。

将上述 9 种注射剂标记好放入 100 ℃ 水浴中加热 1 h，观察溶液颜色随时间的变化。颜色由深至浅分别用 "＋＋＋""＋＋""＋""－" 符号记录，填写于表 3 – 16 中。注射液加热 1 h 后取出，立即用冰水冷却。待注射液温度恢复至室温，测定在 420 nm 处的吸收度，不得超过 0.06。

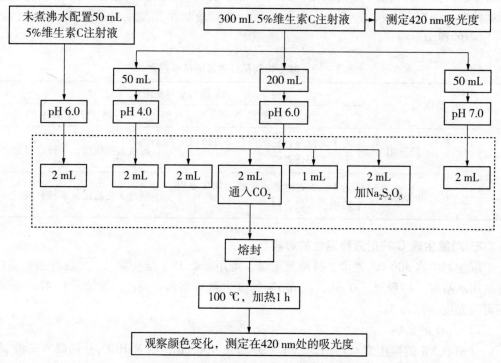

图 3-7　pH 、氧和抗氧剂对维生素 C 注射液稳定性的影响

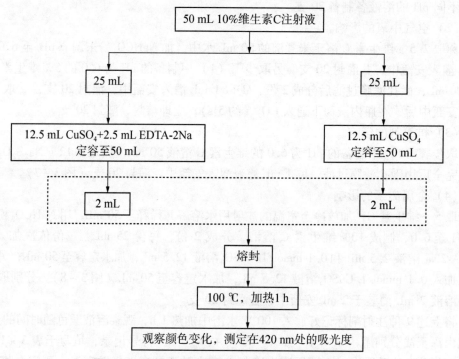

图 3-8　金属离子对维生素 C 注射液稳定性的影响

注意事项

（1）稳定性考察加速实验过程中要注意安全，防止水浴锅烧干导致安瓿爆破伤人。
（2）$NaHCO_3$ 加至维生素 C 溶液中时应缓慢，并充分搅拌。
（3）尽量避免药液与金属器具接触。
（4）选择适合的标记方法，避免加热时由于标记脱落而导致实验失败。

六、实验结果与讨论

（1）维生素 C 注射液的质量检查（表 3 - 14 和表 3 - 15）。

表 3 - 14　注射液装量检查

编号	1	2	3	4	5
实际装量 是否合格					

表 3 - 15　可见异物检查

	初试 20 支	复试 20 支
可见异物数/支 是否合格		

（2）影响维生素 C 注射液稳定性的因素考察（表 3 - 16）。

表 3 - 16　维生素 C 注射液稳定性影响因素考察

样品	样品条件	颜色变化						吸光度 (420 nm)
		0 min	10 min	20 min	30 min	45 min	60 min	
1								
2								
3								
4								
5								
6								
7								
8								
9								

七、思考题

（1）维生素 C 注射液高温加速实验过程中颜色会逐渐加深，最后变成黄色，请解释原因。

（2）制备维生素 C 注射液时通入 CO_2 的目的是什么？

（3）为什么调节 pH 时要缓慢加入 $NaHCO_3$，且要边加边搅拌？

（4）以维生素 C 注射液为例，简述如何筛选注射剂的灭菌条件。

八、常见问题

在采用紫外分光光度计测定吸光度时，应使用配套的比色皿，否则会增加测定的系统误差。

Experiment 4　Preparation of Vitamin C Injections and Investigation on Formulation and Procedure

Ⅰ. Purpose

（1）To master the manufacturing process and key points of preparing injections.

（2）To grasp the quality inspections of injections.

（3）To master the factors that affect the stability of vitamin C injections and various stabilization methods.

（4）To be familiar with the conventional methods measuring the stability of injections.

Ⅱ. Principles

Injections are sterile preparations containing active pharmaceutical ingredients（APIs）and appropriate excipients for parenteral administration into body.

Injections are divided into parenteral solutions, sterile powders and concentrated solutions, etc. Parenteral solutions are sterile liquid preparations including injectable solutions, injectable suspensions and injectable emulsions. According to the routes of administration, injections can be divided into intravenous injections, intramuscular injections, intrathecal injections, intraspinal injections, subcutaneous injections and intradermal injections. Injections are absorbed rapidly *in vivo* and effect quickly as they are administered into tissues or blood vessels of human body directly. In order to ensure the security and efficacy, the manufacturing process and quality injections must be strictly controlled.

The common preparation process of parenteral solutions is shown in Figure 3 − 5:

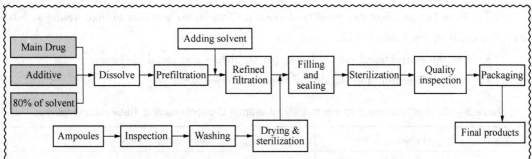

Figure 3 −5   Preparation process of parenteral solutions

The quality inspections of injections include sterility test, bacterial endotoxin test, pyrogen test, visible particles test, pH, filling, osmolality (large-volume injections) and content determination, etc, all of which should comply with requirements within validity period. The pH of injections should be close to physiological pH, generally $4 \sim 9$. The selection of pH depends on the following 3 aspects: firstly, it can satisfy the clinical application; secondly, it should fulfill the demands of the drug stability in preparation, storage and utilization; thirdly, it should possess physiological tolerance. The osmotic pressure of intravenous injection should be isosmotic when dose or dripping infusion in large volume. Drugs unstable in aqueous solution are usually designed as sterile powder to ensure the stability, security and efficacy of the injections within the storage period.

To meet the quality requirements of injections, workshops and operators should meet the GMP requirements during the whole manufacturing process. Drug substances, additives and solvent, etc, must be in line with quality standards for injections. The prescription must adopt the legal prescription, and their preparation methods must strictly abide proposed production procedure rather than get optional change.

The chemical structure of vitamin C (ascorbic acid) is shown in Figure 3 − 6. Two enol groups are easily oxidized under aerobic and anaerobic conditions. There are many factors that affect the stability of vitamin C injections, such as oxygen, pH, metal ions, temperature, light and humidity, etc. The instability of vitamin C mainly reflects in the color change from colorless to yellow and content decrease during

Figure 3 −6   Chemical structure of vitamin C

storage. In addition, the enediol structure of vitamin C lead to the strong acidity and irritating stimulation when injecting. Therefore, both the stability and the tolerance should be fully considered when we design the formulation and procedure of vitamin C injections.

III. Preview

(1) Briefly describe physicochemical properties of vitamin C according to its structural features.

（2）What factors affect the stability of vitamin C injections and how to improve the stability? Please fill in the Table 3 – 12.

（3）List the conventional antioxidants, pH regulators and metal chelators.

（4）How to determine the stability of vitamin C injections?

Table 3 – 12   Factors affecting the stability of vitamin C injections and stabilization methods

Number	Influence factors	Stabilization methods
1		
2		
3		
4		
5		

Ⅳ. Experiment materials and equipments

1. Reagents and experimental materials

Vitamin C, sodium bicarbonate（$NaHCO_3$）, sodium metabisulfite（$Na_2S_2O_5$）, copper sulfate（$CuSO_4$）, edetate disodium（EDTA – 2Na）, methylene blue, water for iniection.

2. Experimental equipments

Ampoule, ultraviolet-visible spectrophotometer, pH meter, water bath, electric stove, ampoule melting and sealing machine, volumetric flask, beaker, clarity detector.

Ⅴ. Experiment contents

1. Preparation of 5% vitamin C injections

1）Prescription：

Vitamin C	2. 50 g
$NaHCO_3$	q. s.
$Na_2S_2O_5$	0. 120 g
EDTA – 2Na	0. 125 g
Water for injections added to	50 mL

2）Procedures：

（1）Treatment of empty ampoules. Wash ampoules twice with regular water and distilled water separately. For contaminated ampoules, add 0. 1% hydrochloric acid into the ampoule, heat for 30 min at 100 ℃ before washing. Dry the clean ampoules at 120 ~ 140 ℃ for the subsequent use.

(2) Preparation of drug solution. EDTA-2Na and vitamin C are dissolved in 40 mL water for injections (boil then cool to room temperature), then $Na_2S_2O_5$ is completely dissolved in the above solution. Add $NaHCO_3$ slowly under stirring until no bubbles produce. Adjust the pH to 5.8 ~ 6.2, and add water for injections to 50 mL.

(3) Perfusion and melting seal. Filter the above solution through 0.22 μm microporous membrane. The filtered solution (2.15 mL) is filled into ampoules. Then seal the ampoules immediately after displacing CO_2 inside the solution and in the container. The instruction of ampoule melting and sealing machine is detailed in Appendix ⅠB.

(4) Sterilization and leakage detection. Sterilize the injections by 100 ℃ in circulating steam for 15 min. Immerse the ampoules in 1% methylene blue solution for leakage check by removing the colored ampoules.

(5) Quality Inspection.

A. Filling. Take 5 containers, open the containers with caution to avoid any loss of the contents. Take up individually the content of each containers into a dry syringe, then discharge the content of syringe into a calibrated cylinder (of such size that volume to be measured occupies at least 40% of its rated volume, do not drain the needle) slowly and continuously. The content in each container should be not less than the labelled quantity.

B. Visible particles inspection. Take 20 containers randomly, remove the adhere labels, clean the outer surface. Hold the bottle-neck of the container at the edge of light shield of the clarity detector (Detailed in Appendix ⅠC), gently swirl and invert the container in order to force the visible particles in the solution being examined floating (ensuring that air bubbles are not introduced). Meanwhile, observe any insoluble substances in the container in front of black background and white background respectively. Repeat several times within 20 s hold 2 containers for each observation. If the air bubbles affect observation, stand until bubbles disappear before examination again. The intensity of illumination should be 1 000 ~ 1 500 lx for examination.

C. Evaluation. The obviously visible impurity particles such as broken bits of metal or glass, fibres with length of more than 2 mm or block with size dimension of more than 2 mm, the smoky precipitate composed by particles formed by gently inverting the container after a period of stationary standing, the cluster of particles which are difficult to count, the precipitate not dispersed on shaking, and the protein flocculus which are difficult to count within the specified time should not be found. If tiny visible particles, such as dots, short fibres or block whose length or size less than 2 mm were found in the containers, they should comply with the requirements listed in Table 3 – 13.

Table 3 –13   Evaluation for non-biological injections

Category		Tiny visible particles limits	
		20 containers for primary test	40 containers in primary and repeat test
Injections	For intravenous	If tiny visible particles have been found in 1 container, repeat the procedure. The number of containers in which tiny visible particles have been found shall be not more than 1	The number of containers in which tiny visible particles have been found shall be not more than 1
	For non-intravenous	If tiny visible particles have been found in 1 or 2 containers, repeat the procedure. The number of containers in which tiny visible particles have been found shall be not more than 2	The number of containers in which tiny visible particles have been found shall be not more than 2

2. Influence of Vitamin C injections

Boil 400 mL of water for injections and then cool to room temperature for later use. Weigh 15 g vitamin C and dissolve in 300 mL of water for injections to prepare 5% vitamin C solutions. Measure the absorbance of vitamin C solution at 420 nm and denote as A_0.

(1) Influence of pH.

Take 50 mL, 200 mL and 50 mL of 5% vitamin C solutions and adjust their pH with NaHCO$_3$ to 4.0, 6.0 and 7.0, respectively. Transfer 2.0 mL of the solution to 2 mL ampoules with a syringe, then seal the ampoule immediately. At last, 20 injections are obtained for each pH.

(2) Influence of oxygen.

Weigh 2.5 g of vitamin C dissolved in 50 mL raw water for injections, adjust the pH to 6.0 with NaHCO$_3$, transfer 2.0 mL to ampoule and seal till 20 injections are obtained in total. In addition, take 100 mL of 5% vitamin C solution with pH 6.0 prepared following step (1), then divide the solutions equally into 2 parts. In one part, transfer 1.0 mL of the solution to 2 mL ampoule and seal, gain 20 injections. In the other part, transfer 2.0 mL of the solution to ampoules, displace the air of the containers only rather than the solution inside by CO$_2$ (about 5 s), and seal the ampoules immediately till gain 20 injections.

(3) Influence of antioxidant.

Take 0.12 g Na$_2$S$_2$O$_5$ dissolved in 50 mL of 5% vitamin C solution with pH 6.0 prepared following step (1). Fill 1.0 mL of the solutions into ampoules and seal, obtain 20 injections in total (Figure 3 –7).

（4）Influence of metal ion.

Take 5 g vitamin C dissolved in 50 mL water for injections to prepare 10% vitamin C solutions, adjust pH to 6.0 with $NaHCO_3$, then divide the solution equally into 2 parts. In one part, add 2.5 mL of 5% EDTA-2Na solution and 12.5 mL of 0.1 mmol/L $CuSO_4$ solution successively, and add water for injections to 50 mL. In the other part, only add 12.5 mL of 0.1 mmol/L $CuSO_4$ solution, and then add water for injections to 50 mL (Figure 3 – 8). Fill 2 mL of the above solutions to 2 mL ampoules and seal, and gain 20 injections, respectively.

Label the above 9 prescriptions of vitamin C injections and heat for 1 h at 100 ℃ in a water bath. Observe the color change of the solutions with time, and record the color change with " + + + " " + + " " + " " – " from dark to light, and fill them in Table 3 – 16. After heating for 1 h, cool the injections to room temperature in an ice-water bath immediately. Measure the absorbance at 420 nm, and the absorbance should not exceed 0.06.

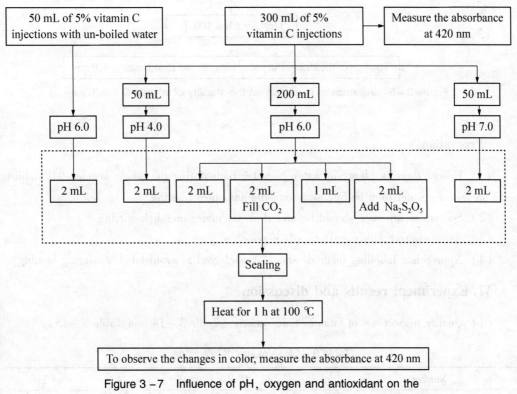

Figure 3 – 7　Influence of pH, oxygen and antioxidant on the
stability of vitamin C injections

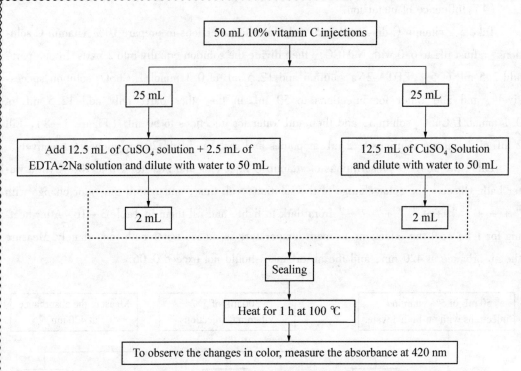

Figure 3 −8   Influence of metal ion on the stability of vitamin C injections

[**Precautions**]

(1) Ensure there is plenty of water in water bath during the whole accelerated stability test, prevent the water from boiling away causing ampoules blasting.

(2) Sodium bicarbonate should be added slowly under thorough stirring.

(3) Avoid contact with metal utensils if possible.

(4) Appropriate labelling methods should be selected to avoid label-off during heating.

VI. Experiment results and discussion

(1) Quality inspections of vitamin C injections (Table 3 −14 and Table 3 −15).

Table 3 −14   Volume of injections

Number	1	2	3	4	5
Actual volume of injections					
Qualified or not					

Table 3 – 15   Test for visible particles

	20 containers for primary test	20 containers for repeat test
The number of containers in which tiny visible particles have been found		
Qualified or not		

(2) Inspecting the factors affecting the stability of vitamin C injections (Table 3 – 16).

Table 3 – 16   Factors affecting the stability of vitamin C injections

Sample	Sample condition	Color change						Absorbance (at 420 nm)
		0 min	10 min	20 min	30 min	45 min	60 min	
1								
2								
3								
4								
5								
6								
7								
8								
9								

VII. Questions

(1) During the accelerated stability test, the color of vitamin C injections gradually deepen and eventually turn yellow. Explain it.

(2) Why CO_2 is used in vitamin C injections preparation?

(3) Why is sodium bicarbonate added slowly under thorough stirring when adjusting pH ?

(4) How to screen the sterilization condition of injections? Take vitamin C injection as an example.

VIII. Common questions

When using ultraviolet spectrophotometer to measure the absorbance, matched cuvettes should be used to attenuate the system error.

实验五　颗粒剂的制备

一、实验目的

（1）掌握颗粒剂的干法制粒和湿法制粒制备方法。
（2）掌握颗粒剂常用附加剂。
（3）熟悉颗粒剂的质量检查方法。

二、实验原理

颗粒剂（granules）系指药物与适宜的辅料混合制成具有一定粒度的干燥颗粒状制剂。颗粒剂主要供口服给药，既可吞服，又可混悬或溶解在水中服用。根据其在水中的溶解情况，可分为可溶颗粒剂、混悬颗粒剂和泡腾颗粒剂。根据释放行为的不同，可分为速释颗粒剂、肠溶颗粒剂、缓控释颗粒剂等。

颗粒剂具有服用方便、吸收迅速、起效快等特点。通过制粒，可减少粉末飞散、附着和团聚（与散剂相比），同时增加粉体的流动性。颗粒剂的制备方法分为干法制粒和湿法制粒。湿法制粒的工艺流程如图 3 - 9 所示：将药物与辅料混合后，加黏合剂或润湿剂制软材，制粒、干燥、整粒后分装即得。其中，粉碎、过筛、混合是保证固体药物含量均匀度的主要操作单元。

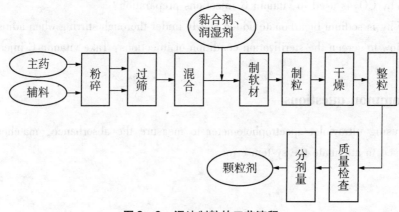

图 3 - 9　湿法制粒的工艺流程

粉碎（crushing），是指借助机械力将大块的固体物质粉碎成合适粒径的操作过程。根据物料的性质，粉碎方法可分为干法粉碎、湿法粉碎、低温粉碎和超微粉碎等。过筛（sieving），是指利用具有不同尺寸筛孔的筛子对固体物料进行分离的操作。可通过电动筛、分样筛及旋风分离器等实现。混合（mixing），是指两种或多种物料相互分散而达到一定均匀程度的单元操作，混合方法可分为搅拌混合、研磨混合、过筛混合。

制软材为湿法制粒的关键步骤，软材应以"轻握成团，轻压即散"为度。

颗粒剂的质量检查项目除外观与含量测定外，还包括粒度、干燥失重、水分（中药颗粒剂）、溶化性和装量差异等。

三、预习思考

（1）具备什么特点的药物适合设计成颗粒剂？

（2）根据颗粒剂的分类，列举 1～2 种市售颗粒剂，阐述其剂型设计依据。

四、实验材料与仪器

1. 实验试剂与试药

维生素 C、对乙酰氨基酚、乳酸菌素、酒石酸、日落黄、碳酸氢钠、氯化钠、蔗糖、阿司帕坦、羟丙甲纤维素（50 cp）、糊精、淀粉、甘露醇、糖粉、二氧化硅、乙醇、枸橼酸、五氧化二磷、醋酸、碘滴定液、淀粉指示剂、蒸馏水。

2. 实验仪器

电炉、筛网、烧杯、烘箱、热封机、喷雾器、天平、溶出度仪、紫外分光光度计。

五、实验内容

（一）对乙酰氨基酚颗粒剂（可溶颗粒剂）

1. 处方

对乙酰氨基酚	10 g
糊精	30 g
淀粉	60 g
10% 淀粉浆	适量

2. 实验步骤

（1）称取淀粉约 4 g，在 40 mL 蒸馏水中分散均匀，加热糊化（80～85 ℃），得 10% 淀粉浆。

（2）按处方量将对乙酰氨基酚、糊精和淀粉分别过 100 目筛，混合均匀。再加适量 10% 淀粉浆制软材，挤压过 16 目筛。

（3）湿颗粒于 60 ℃干燥，过 16 目筛整粒。

（4）测定颗粒中对乙酰氨基酚的含量，按 0.1 g 标示量分装，密封即得。

3. 质量检查

（1）粒度：照粒度和粒度分布测定法（2020 版《中国药典》通则 0982 第二法），取供试品 5 袋，称定质量，置上层一号筛中（下层的五号筛下配有密合的接收容器），保持水平状态过筛，左右往返，边筛动边拍打 3 min。不能通过一号筛与能通过五号筛的总和不得超过 15%。

（2）干燥失重：照干燥失重测定法（2020 版《中国药典》通则 0831）测定，于 105 ℃干燥至恒重，减失质量不得超过 2.0%。

（3）溶出度：取供试品 6 袋（瓶），照 2020 版《中国药典》溶出度与释放度测定法（通则 0931 第二法），分别以稀盐酸 24 mL 加水至 1 000 mL 为溶出介质，转速为 50 r/min 转，依法操作 30 min 后，取溶液 10 mL，滤过，精密量取续滤液适量，用 0.04% 氢氧化钠溶液稀释制成每毫升中含对乙酰氨基酚约 8 μg 的溶液，依照紫外 – 可见分光光度法（通则 0401），在 257 nm 的波长处测定吸光度，按 $C_8H_9NO_2$ 的吸收系数 $E_{1\,cm}^{1\%}$ 为 715 计算每袋（瓶）的溶出量，限度为标示量的 80%，应符合规定。

（4）装量差异：照颗粒剂项下装量差异检查法（2020 版《中国药典》通则 0104），取供试品 10 袋，除去包装，分别精密称定每袋内容物的质量，每袋装量与标示装量比较，超出装量差异限度的颗粒剂不得多于 2 袋（瓶），并不得有 1 袋超出装量差异限度 1 倍，装量差异限度要求见表 3 – 17。

表 3 – 17　装量差异限度

平均装量或标示装量	装量差异限度
1.0 g 及以下	±10%
1.0 g 以上至 1.5 g	±8%
1.5 g 以上至 6.0 g	±7%
6.0 g 以上	±5%

（二）乳酸菌素颗粒剂（混悬颗粒剂）

1. 处方

乳酸菌素	50 g
甘露醇	15 g
糖粉	15 g
淀粉	11 g
二氧化硅	3.0 g
阿司帕坦	4.5 g
80% 乙醇	适量

2. 实验步骤

（1）将乳酸菌素、糖粉、淀粉和二氧化硅等辅料过 100 目筛，混合均匀。

（2）80% 乙醇用喷雾器以雾状喷入上述混合物中，制软材，挤压过 16 目筛。

（3）湿颗粒于 45 ℃ 以下干燥，过 16 目筛整粒。

（4）测定乳酸菌素含量，按 1.0 g 标示量分装，密封即得。

3. 质量检查

（1）粒度及装量差异参照对乙酰氨基酚颗粒剂。

（2）干燥失重：取本品，以五氧化二磷为干燥剂，60 ℃ 减压干燥至恒重，减失质量不得超过 5.0%。

注意事项

（1）减压干燥时，除另有规定外压力应在 2.67 kPa（20 mmHg）以下。

（2）生物制品除另有规定外，减压干燥温度为 60 ℃。

（3）测定溶出度时，颗粒剂应在溶出介质表面分散投样，避免集中投样。

（4）混悬型颗粒剂无须进行溶化性检查。

（三）维生素 C 泡腾颗粒剂（泡腾颗粒剂）

1. 处方

（1）酸粒：

维生素 C	15 g
酒石酸	105 g
日落黄	0.1 g

（2）碱粒：

碳酸氢钠	120 g
氯化钠	3.0 g
蔗糖	40 g
阿司帕坦	5.0 g
日落黄	1.0 g
羟丙甲纤维素	5.0 g

2. 实验步骤

（1）将维生素 C 和辅料分别过 100 目筛。

（2）酸粒的制备：将处方量日落黄通过超声溶于适量的 80% 乙醇溶液中，得到含有色素的乙醇溶液。将维生素 C、酒石酸按处方量混合均匀后，用配好的含有色素的乙醇溶液制备软材，过 16 目筛制粒，50 ℃烘干，16 目筛整粒。

（3）碱粒的制备：将日落黄溶于 5% 的羟丙甲纤维素（50 cp）溶液中，得到黄色黏合剂溶液。将碳酸氢钠、氯化钠及蔗糖按处方量混合均匀后，加入黏合剂制备软材，过 16 目筛制粒，50 ℃烘干，16 目筛整粒。

（4）将上述酸粒与碱粒按处方比例混合，测定颗粒中维生素 C 的含量，按 0.2 g 标示量分装，密封即得。

3. 质量检查

（1）粒度、装量差异和干燥失重检查参照对乙酰氨基酚颗粒剂。

（2）酸度：取本品 7.5 g，加水 100 mL，待溶解完全无气泡后，照 pH 测定法（2020 版《中国药典》通则 0631）测定 pH，pH 应为 4.5～5.5。

（3）溶化性：照泡腾颗粒检查法（2020 版《中国药典》通则 0104），取供试品 3 袋，将内容物分别转移至盛有 200 mL 水的烧杯中，水温为 15～25 ℃，应迅速产生气体而呈泡腾状，5 min 内颗粒均应完全分散或溶解在水中，且不得有异物。

（4）含量测定：取装量差异项下的内容物，混合均匀，精密称取适量（约相当于 0.2 g 维生素 C），加新煮沸过的冷水 100 mL 与稀醋酸 10 mL 使维生素 C 溶解，加淀粉指示液 1 mL，立即用碘滴定液（0.05 mol/L）滴定，至溶液显蓝色并持续 30 s 不褪色。每毫升碘滴定液（0.05 mol/L）相当于 8.806 mg 的 $C_6H_8O_6$。

4. 酸源种类及用量对维生素 C 泡腾颗粒剂质量的影响

保持维生素 C 泡腾颗粒剂其他组分不变，改变酒石酸用量分别为 70 g、105 g 和 140 g，制备泡腾颗粒剂，测定三种颗粒剂的 pH 和溶化性。

保持泡腾颗粒剂中其他组分不变，将酒石酸换成枸橼酸，制备泡腾颗粒剂，比较两种酸源制备的颗粒剂的 pH 和溶化时限。

注意事项

制粒过程应避免接触金属，并尽量缩短制粒时间。

六、实验结果与讨论

1. 颗粒剂的质量检查结果

将测得的结果填入表 3 - 18 ～ 表 3 - 21。

表 3 - 18　颗粒剂的质量检查

外观	粒度/%	干燥失重/%	pH	含量/%

表3-19　溶出度检查结果

编号	1	2	3	4	5	6	平均值
溶出量/mg							
溶出度/%							
结论							

表3-20　装量差异检查结果

编号	1	2	3	4	5	6	7	8	9	10	标示量/g
装量/g											
装量差异/%											
结论											

表3-21　溶化性检查结果

编号	1	2	3
溶化时限/s			
结论			

2. 酸源种类及用量对维生素 C 泡腾颗粒剂质量的影响

将测得的结果填入表3-22。

表3-22　不同处方维生素 C 泡腾颗粒剂的 pH 和溶化时限

酸源种类及用量	pH	溶化时限/s	结论
70 g 酒石酸			
105 g 酒石酸			
140 g 酒石酸			
105 g 枸橼酸			

七、思考题

（1）上述三种颗粒剂的质量检查项目有何不同？

（2）不同类型颗粒剂其干燥失重的测定方法有何不同？请依 2020 版《中国药典》（通则 0831）加以解释。

Experiment 5　Preparation of Granules

I. Purpose

（1）To master preparation methods of dry granulation and wet granulation.

（2）To know different types of conventional additives used in granules.

（3）To be familiar with the quality inspections of granules.

II. Principles

Granules are dry granular preparations with appropriate particle size made of drug substances and suitable excipients. Granules, mainly for oral administration, can be taken by swallowing or dissolving/suspending in water. It can be divided into soluble granules, suspended granules and effervescent granules based on its solubility in water; or divided into immediate-release granules, enteric-coated granules, sustained-release granules and controlled-release granules according to its drug release behavior.

Granules have the characteristics of easy taking, fast absorption *in vivo* and fast onset. Granulating can lower the dispersion, adhesion and agglomeration rate of powder with higher fluidity (compared with powder). Preparation methods of granules are generally divided into dry granulation and wet granulation. The wet granulation process is shown in Figure 3 – 9. After mixing the active substances and excipients, add adhesive or wetting agents to prepare soft materials, and subsequently granulate and dry granules, then subpackage to obtain the final granules. Crushing, sieving and mixing are the main operation units to ensure the uniformity of drug content.

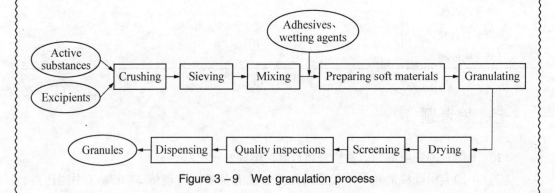

Figure 3 – 9　Wet granulation process

Crushing is the process of pressing large solid materials into a suitable size by means of mechanical force. According to the properties of materials, crushing methods can be divided into dry crushing, wet crushing, low temperature crushing and ultrafine crushing, etc. Sieving is a technique for separating particles of different sizes by using sieves (electric sieve, sample sieve or cyclone separator, etc.). Mixing is a unit operation that involves manipulation of two or more materials to make them into a certain uniformity. Mixing methods can be divided into stirring mixing, grinding mixing and sieving mixing.

Preparation of soft materials is a key step of wet granulation, which should be done with "gripped into clumps, pressed to spallation but not fragmented in powder".

The quality inspections of granules include determination of appearance and content, particle size, loss on drying, determination of water (for Chinese medicinal granules), dispersion, weight variation.

Ⅲ. Preview

(1) What kind of drugs are suitable to be formulated as granules?

(2) According to the classification of granules, list $1 \sim 2$ kinds of commercially available granules and illustrate the thought of dosage form design.

Ⅳ. Experiment materials and equipments

1. Reagents and experimental materials

Vitamin C, acetaminophen, lactein, tartaric acid, sunset yellow, sodium bicarbonate, sodium chloride, sucrose, aspartame, hypromellose (50 cp), dextrin, starch, mannitol, powdered sugar, silicon, dioxide ethanol, citric acid, phosphorus pentoxide, acetic acid, iodine titration solution, starch indicator, distilled water.

2. Experimental equipments

Electric stove, sieve, beaker, drying oven, heat sealer, sprayer, balance, dissolution apparatus, UV spectrophotometer.

Ⅴ. Experiment contents

1. Acetaminophen granules (soluble granules)

1) Formulation:

Acetaminophen	10 g
Dextrin	30 g
Starch	60 g
10% starch paste	q. s.

2) Procedures:

(1) Weigh about 4 g of starch and disperse it in 40 mL distilled water, and heat the mixture in a water bath at $80 \sim 85$ ℃ for gelatinization to obtain 10% of starch paste.

(2) Pass acetaminophen, dextrin and starch through a 100-mesh sieve, respectively. Then

mix them evenly and add an appropriate amount of 10% starch paste to prepare soft materials, then squeeze soft materials through a 16-mesh sieve for granulation.

(3) Dry wet granules at 60 ℃, then pass them through a 16-mesh sieve.

(4) Determine the content of acetaminophen in granules, pack granules with the labeled amount of 0. 1 g, and seal them to obtain final granules.

3) Quality inspections.

(1) Particle size:

According to the Determination of Particle Size and Particle Size Distribution [0982 of method 2, *Chinese pharmacopoeia* 2020 edition (ChP 2020)], take 5 packs of granules, weigh and put granules in the upper layer No. 1 sieve (the No. 5 sieve on the lower layer shall be equipped with a hermetic receiving container). Keep sieve in a horizontal state, shift back and forth, and tap while sieving for 3 min. The total weight of granules which can not pass through No. 1 sieve but can pass through NO. 5 sieve should not be more than 15% of the test samples.

(2) Loss on drying:

According to the method for Loss on Drying (0831, ChP 2020), dry the samples to constant weight at 105 ℃, and the weight loss should not be more than 2. 0%.

(3) Dissolution:

This process shall be operated according to the method for dissolution and release determination (method 2, 0931, ChP 2020). Dilute 24 mL hydrochloric acid into 1 000 mL water to prepare dissolution medium, then add granules into dissolution medium, rotate the solution at a rotation speed of 50 r/min for 30 min. Then take 10 mL of the solution, filter it, and precisely take an appropriate amount of the filtrate. Dilute the filtrate with 0. 04% sodium hydroxide solution to make the solution with the concentration of acetaminophen is about 8 μg/mL. Then comply with the method for ultraviolet-visible spectrophotometry (0401, ChP 2020), measure the absorbance at 257 nm, and calculate the amount of acetaminophen dissolved from each packet given that the absorptivity $E_{1\text{ cm}}^{1\%}$ of $C_8H_9NO_2$ is 715. The value of quantity is required to be higher than 80% of the labelled content.

(4) Weight variation:

According to weight variation test (0104, ChP 2020), take 10 packs of the granules, discard the wrapper, and accurately weigh the content of each separately. Compare the weight of each pack with the labelled weight. No more than 2 individual values should deviate more than the limit, and none should deviate more than twice the limit. Weight variation limit should comply with the requirements listed in Table 3 – 17.

Table 3 –17 Limits for granule weight variation

Average or labelled weight	Weight variation limit
1. 0 g or less	±10%
1. 0 g to 1. 5 g	±8%
1. 5 g to 6. 0 g	±7%
Above 6. 0 g	±5%

2. Preparation of lactein granules (suspended granules)

1) Formulation:

Lactein	50 g
Mannitol	15 g
Powdered sugar	15 g
Starch	11 g
Silica	3. 0 g
Aspartame	4. 5 g
80% ethanol	q. s.

2) Procedures:

(1) Pass lactein, powdered sugar, starch and silicon dioxide through a 100-mesh sieve respectively and then mix them thoroughly.

(2) Spray 80% ethanol into the mixture obtained above to prepare soft materials, and screen the soft materials through a 16-mesh sieve to obtain wet granules.

(3) Dry wet granules below 45 ℃, and press them through a 16-mesh sieve.

(4) Determine the content of lactein, pack granules with 1 g labeled amount, and seal them to obtain final granules.

3) Quality inspections:

(1) Particle size and weight variation tests refer to those of acetaminophen granules.

(2) Loss on drying. Take the lactein granules and dry under reduced pressure to constant weight at 60 ℃ with phosphorus pentoxide as the desiccant. Weight loss should not be more than 5. 0%.

[Precautions]

(1) Unless otherwise specified, pressure should be below 2. 67 kPa (20 mmHg) when drying under reduced pressure.

(2) Unless otherwise specified, reduced pressure drying temperature for biological products should be 60 ℃.

（3）When measuring the dissolution, the granules should be scattered on the surface of dissolution medium to avoid concentrated sample-adding.

（4）Dispersion test is not necessity for suspended granules.

3. Preparation of vitamin C effervescent granules（effervescent granules）

1）Formulation：

（1）Acid granules：

Vitamin C	15 g
Tartaric acid	105 g
Sunset yellow	0.1 g

（2）Alkali granules：

Sodium bicarbonate	120 g
Sodium chloride	3.0 g
Sucrose	40 g
Aspartame	5.0 g
Sunset yellow	1.0 g
Hypromellose	5.0 g

2）Procedures：

（1）Pass vitamin C and excipients through a 100-mesh sieve respectively.

（2）Preparation of acid granules：dissolve sunset yellow by ultrasonication in an appropriate amount of 80% ethanol to obtain ethanol solution containing pigment. After mixing vitamin C and tartaric acid, add ethanol solution containing pigment to make soft materials, pass the soft materials through a 16-mesh sieve for granulation. Dry granules at 50 ℃, and pass dry granules through a 16-mesh sieve.

（3）Preparation of alkali granules：dissolve sunset yellow in a 5% hypromellose solution （50 cp）to obtain yellow binder solution. Mix sodium bicarbonate, sodium chloride and sucrose, then add binder solution to make soft materials, pass the soft materials through a 16-mesh sieve for granulation. Dry granules at 50 ℃, and pass dry granules through a 16-mesh sieve.

（4）Mix the above acid granules and alkali granules, determine the content of vitamin C, pack granules with 0.2 g labeled amount, and seal them to obtain final granules.

3）Quality inspections：

（1）Particle size, weight variation and loss on drying inspection should refer to those of acetaminophen granules.

（2）Acidity：take 7.5 g granules and dissolve them in 100 mL of distilled water. After dissolving completely without bubbles, comply with the method for pH measurement (0631, ChP 2020) to measure pH. The range of pH should be 4.5～5.5.

(3) Dispersion: according to the Dispersion Test for effervescent granules (0104 Granules, ChP 2020), take 3 packs of test samples and transfer them to a 250 mL breaker containing 200 mL of 15～25 ℃ water. Bubbles of effervescent appearance should generate at once. Granules should disperse completely or dissolve in the water within 5 min, and there must be no foreign matter.

(4) Content determination: take granulations under weight variation test, mix them thoroughly, weigh accurately the appropriate amount (equivalent to about 0.2 g vitamin C), dissolve them in 100 mL of freshly boiled cold water and 10 mL of dilute acetic acid, add 1 mL of starch indicator solution, titrate with iodine titration solution (0.05 mol/L) immediately until the solution color turns to blue and does not fade in 30 s. One milliliter of iodine titration solution (0.05 mol/L) should equal to 8.806 mg of $C_6H_8O_6$.

4. Effects of acid source types and doses on the quality of vitamin C effervescent granules

Keep the content of other components in vitamin C effervescent granules the same, adjust the dose of tartaric acid to 70 g, 105 g and 140 g respectively and prepare effervescent granules, then determine the pH and dispersion of three granules.

Keep other components in the effervescent granules the same, replace the tartaric acid with citric acid, prepare effervescent granules, then compare pH and dispersion of 2 types granules prepared by two acid sources.

[Precautions]

Avoid contacting any metal during the granulation process and shorten the granulation time as possible.

VI. Experiment results and discussion

1. Quality inspections results of granules

Fill the results in Table 3 – 18 to Table 3 – 21.

Table 3 – 18　Quality inspections of granules

Appearance	Particle size/%	Loss on drying/%	pH	Content/%

Table 3 – 19   Dissolution

Number	1	2	3	4	5	6	Average
The amount of drug dissolved/mg							
Dissolution percentage/%							
Conclusion							

Table 3 – 20   Weight variation

Number	1	2	3	4	5	6	7	8	9	10	Labelled weight/g
Weight/g											
Weight variation/%											
Conclusion											

Table 3 – 21   Dispersion

Number	1	2	3
Dispersion time/s			
Conclusion			

2. Effects of acid source types and doses on the quality of vitamin C effervescent granules
Fill the results in Table 3 – 22.

Table 3 – 22   pH and dispersion time of different vitamin C effervescent granules

Acid source types and doses	pH	Dispersion time/s	Conclusion
70 g tartaric acid			
105 g tartaric acid			
140 g tartaric acid			
105 g citric acid			

VII. Questions

(1) What are the differences in quality inspections of three kinds of granules?

(2) Please illustrate the differences in determination methods of loss on drying for different kinds of granules (0831, ChP 2020).

实验六　　硬胶囊剂的制备

一、实验目的

（1）掌握硬胶囊剂的一般制备工艺。
（2）熟悉硬胶囊剂的装量差异检查方法。

二、实验原理

　　胶囊剂（capsules）系指将药物与适宜辅料填装于硬质空心胶囊或有弹性的软质空胶囊中制成的固体制剂。填装于硬质空心胶囊的被称为硬胶囊剂（hard capsules）；填装于有弹性的软质空胶囊的被称为软胶囊剂（soft capsules）。根据药物释放速度和部位的不同可以将胶囊剂设计成缓控释胶囊或肠溶胶囊等。胶囊剂主要供口服用，也可供直肠、阴道使用。硬胶囊剂的空心胶囊主要材料为明胶，也可用甲基纤维素、海藻酸盐类、聚乙烯醇、变性明胶及其他高分子材料。空心胶囊呈圆筒状，是由帽与体两节套合而成的、质硬且有弹性的囊，分透明、半透明与不透明三种类型；根据锁扣类型，分为普通型与锁口型两类；根据规格从大到小分为 000 号、00 号、0 号、1 号、2 号、3 号、4 号、5 号等 8 种，常用 0～5 号。

　　硬胶囊剂的内容物通常是固态，也可以是半固态，可根据药物性质和临床需要制备成不同形式的内容物，主要分为粉末、颗粒和微丸。

　　大量生产时可用全自动胶囊填充机进行药物填充，填充好的药物使用胶囊抛光机直接去除粉尘，提高胶囊光洁度。小量试制可用胶囊填充板或手工填充药物，填充好的胶囊可用喷有少许液状石蜡的纱布轻搓，去除粉尘的同时提高胶囊的光洁度。制备好的胶囊用铝塑包装机包装或装入适宜的容器中。胶囊剂须进行外观、装量差异、崩解时限/溶出度、微生物限度等项目的检查，中药硬胶囊剂还应进行水分检查。

三、预习思考

（1）哪些药物适合设计成胶囊剂？
（2）哪些药物不适于设计成胶囊剂？
（3）空心胶囊规格的选择依据是什么？

四、实验材料与仪器

1. 实验试剂与试药

延胡索浸膏、白芷、对乙酰氨基酚、维生素 C、胆汁粉、咖啡因、氯苯那敏、阿司匹林、滑石粉、淀粉、食用色素、液状石蜡、空胶囊、蒸馏水。

2. 实验仪器

研钵、玻璃板、天平、烧杯、量筒、玻璃棒、胶囊填充板、100 目筛、80 目筛、14目尼龙筛、恒温水浴锅、崩解仪。

五、实验内容

（一）元胡止痛胶囊（手工填充法）

1. 处方

延胡索浸膏	5 g
白芷	20 g
淀粉	25 g
滑石粉	0.5 g
共制成	100 粒

2. 实验步骤

（1）淀粉干燥，过 100 目筛。

（2）将延胡索浸膏和白芷粉分别粉碎，过 100 目筛。

（3）先将药粉混合均匀，再加干淀粉混合均匀，最后加入滑石粉充分混匀。

（4）将混匀粉末置于洁净的玻璃板上，用药匙铺平并压紧，厚度约为胶囊体高度的 1/4 或 1/3。手持胶囊壳，口垂直向下插入粉末，使药粉压入胶囊内，同法操作数次，至每粒胶囊填装 0.30 g 的药粉，套上囊帽。

（5）套囊帽时，先将囊帽口内侧一边紧贴囊体口，然后套入，可避免囊帽切开囊体，套帽时用力宜均匀。

注意事项

（1）药粉与淀粉应充分混合，避免混合不均导致胶囊剂药物含量出现差异。

（2）填充过程中施压应均匀，并注意随时称重以确保胶囊装量准确。

（3）为保证胶囊剂外形光洁，可用喷有少许液状石蜡的洁净纱布轻轻滚搓，拭去胶囊剂表面黏附的药粉。

（二）阿司匹林胶囊（板装法）

1. 处方

阿司匹林	200 g
淀粉	200 g
滑石粉	8 g
共制成	1 000 粒

2. 实验步骤

（1）淀粉干燥，过 100 目筛。

（2）阿司匹林粉碎，过 100 目筛。

（3）将阿司匹林与淀粉混匀，再加入滑石粉混匀。

（4）将 1 号胶囊体插入胶囊板中（使用说明详见附录 ID），将混匀后的药粉置于胶囊填充板上，轻轻敲动胶囊板，至药粉全部均匀填装入胶囊壳中，套上胶囊帽，即得。

（三）速效感冒胶囊（板装法）

1. 处方

对乙酰氨基酚	300 g
维生素 C	100 g
胆汁粉	100 g
咖啡因	3 g
氯苯那敏	3 g
10% 淀粉浆	适量
食用色素	适量
共制成	1 000 粒

2. 实验步骤

（1）取上述各药物，分别粉碎，过 80 目筛。

（2）称取淀粉约 10 g，加入 100 mL 蒸馏水中分散均匀，加热糊化（80～85 ℃），得 10% 淀粉浆。冷却后将其分为 3 份，按 A、B、C 字母顺序进行编号：A 中加入少量食用胭脂红制成红糊；B 中加入少量食用橘黄（最大用量为万分之一）制成黄糊；C 中不加色素制成白糊。

（3）将对乙酰氨基酚分为 3 份：1 份与氯苯那敏混匀后加入红糊；1 份与胆汁粉、维生素 C 混匀后加入黄糊；1 份与咖啡因混匀后加入白糊。分别制成软材后，过 14 目尼龙筛制粒，于70 ℃干燥至水分含量小于3%。

（4）将3种颗粒充分混合至颜色均匀。

（5）将胶囊体插入胶囊板中（使用说明详见附录ID），然后取混合颗粒置于胶囊填充板上，轻轻敲动胶囊板，至药物颗粒全部均匀填装入胶囊壳中，套上胶囊帽。

注意事项

（1）速效感冒胶囊为复方制剂，且处方中药物含量较为悬疏，为避免由于含量和密度差异导致药物混合不均，以及填充时出现离析现象，本实验采取制粒后填充胶囊的策略，以增加药物混合的均一性和粉体的流动性，利于胶囊填充。

（2）由于3种颗粒混合前呈现3种颜色，故可通过观察颜色的均一性来判断颗粒混合的均匀度。

六、实验结果与讨论

对胶囊剂进行外观、水分、装量差异和崩解时限检查。

1. 外观

胶囊剂应整洁，不得有黏结、变形、渗漏或囊壳破裂等现象，应无异臭。

2. 水分

中药硬胶囊剂应进行水分检查。取供试品内容物，照水分测定法（2020版《中国药典》通则0832）测定。除另有规定外，不得超过9.0%。

3. 装量差异

除另有规定外，取供试品20粒（中药取10粒），分别精密称定质量，倾出内容物（不得损失囊壳），硬胶囊囊壳用小刷或其他适宜的用具拭净，再分别精密称定囊壳质量，求出每粒内容物的装量与平均装量。每粒装量与平均装量相比较（有标示装量的胶囊剂，每粒装量应与标示装量比较），超出装量差异限度的不得多于2粒，并不得有1粒超出限度1倍（表3-23）。将测得的结果填入表3-24。

表3-23　胶囊剂装量差异限度

平均装量	装量差异限度
0.30 g以下	±10%
0.30 g及以上	±7.5%

表3-24 胶囊剂装量差异检查结果

编号	胶囊重量/g	囊壳重量/g	内容物装量/g	编号	胶囊重量/g	囊壳重量/g	内容物装量/g
1				11			
2				12			
3				13			
4				14			
5				15			
6				16			
7				17			
8				18			
9				19			
10				20			
平均装量/g							
装量限度/g							
是否合格							

4. 崩解时限

除另有规定外，取供试品6粒，用崩解仪测定硬胶囊剂崩解时限，若胶囊剂漂浮在液面，可加1块挡板。硬胶囊应在30 min内全部崩解。如有1粒不能完全崩解，应另取6粒复试，均应符合规定。凡规定检查溶出度或释放度的胶囊剂可不再进行崩解时限检查。

七、思考题

（1）在元胡止痛胶囊处方中，滑石粉和淀粉的作用分别是什么？
（2）评价粉体流动性的指标有哪些？

Experiment 6　Preparation of Hard Capsules

Ⅰ. Purpose

（1）To master the preparation process of hard capsules.
（2）To be familiar with weight variation test of hard capsules.

Ⅱ. Principles

Capsules are solid pharmaceutical dosage forms in which active pharmaceutical ingredients（APIs）and excipients are enclosed in hollow hard capsules or soft shells. Capsules are divided into hard capsules and soft capsules according to the materials of capsule shells. They can also be classified into sustained-release capsules and enteric-coated capsules according to release rate and action site of drugs. Capsules are mainly used for oral administration, and also for rectal and vaginal administration. The shells of hard capsules are usually made from gelatin, and may also be made from methylcellulose, alginate, polyvinyl alcohol, denatured gelatin and so on. The empty capsule shell is a hard and elastic container consisting of a cap-piece interlocking with a body-piece. They can be divided into transparent capsules, translucent capsules and opaque capsules based on their appearance, ordinary capsules and coni-snap capsules according to the lock type, or classified into No. 000, No. 00, No. 0, No. 1, No. 2, No. 3, No. 4, and No. 5 according to their size from large to small. Among them, size from No. 0 to No. 5 are commonly used.

The contents of hard capsules are usually solid or semi-solid in form. The contents of hard capsules may be powders, granules or pellets according to drug properties and clinical needs.

Different methods are adopted for filling capsules. For mass production, the automatic capsule filling machine is used. The filled hard capsules can be directly dedusted, cleaned, and polished by the capsule-polishing machine. For a small amount of lab-scale preparation, manual filling is carried out including by means of capsule filling plates. The filled capsules can be dedusted, cleaned, and polished by gently wiping with a gauze with little liquid paraffin. Once ready, those filled and dedusted capsules shall be packaged with the aluminum-plastic packaging machine or filled in a suitable container. Quality inspections of capsules including appearance, weight variation, disintegration/dissolution, and microbial limit will be conducted. And water determination is required for Chinese medicine hard capsules.

Ⅲ. Preview

(1) What kinds of drugs are suitable to be designed as capsules?

(2) What kinds of drugs are not suitable to be formulated as capsules?

(3) What is the basis to choose the size of empty capsules?

Ⅳ. Experiment materials and equipments

1. Reagents and experimental materials

Corydalis extract, angelica dahurica, acetaminophen, vitamin C, bile powder, caffeine, chlorpheniramine, aspirin, talcum powder, starch, food colorant, liquid paraffin, empty capsules and distilled water.

2. Experimental equipments

Mortar, glass plate, balance, beaker, measuring cylinder, glass rod, capsule filling plate, 100-mesh sieve, 80-mesh sieve, 14-mesh nylon sieve, thermostatic water bath, and disintegration instrument.

V. Experiment content

1. Analgesic capsule of corydalis tuber (Manual filling)

1) Formulation:

Corydalis extract	5 g
Angelica dahurica	20 g
Starch	25 g
Talcum powder	0.5 g
Obtain	100 capsules

2) Procedures:

(1) Pass the dried starch through 100-mesh sieve.

(2) Grind the corydalis extract and angelica dahurica separately, then pass them through 100-mesh sieve.

(3) Mix the powder of two drugs thoroughly, and add the dry starch and mix thoroughly. Finally add talcum powder and mix thoroughly.

(4) Place mixed powder on a clean glass plate, flatten and compress it with a spatula to make a solid mixture layer about 1/4 to 1/3 of a capsule's height in thickness. Hold the capsule shell body, insert into the powder vertically downwards to press the powder into the capsules. Operate for several times in the same way until each capsule is filled with 0.30 g of mixed powder, then put the cap on it.

(5) When putting the cap on, firstly ensure the inner side of the cap tightly attached to the mouth of the body to avoid the body being cut into pieces. The process should be handled carefully with even force.

[Precautions]

(1) Mix the drugs and starch thoroughly to avoid drug content difference unqualified.

(2) Press the powder evenly during the filling process, and weigh the capsules at any needed time to ensure an accurate loading weight.

(3) To ensure the smooth and cleanness of capsules, a clean gauze sprayed with a little liquid paraffin can be used to wipe off drug powders adhering to the surface of capsules.

2. Aspirin capsules (plate filling)

1) Formulation:

Aspirin	200 g
Starch	200 g
Talcum powder	8 g
Obtain	1 000 capsules

2) Procedures:

(1) Pass the dried starch through 100-mesh sieve.

(2) Grind aspirin and passed it through the 100-mesh sieve.

(3) Mix aspirin and starch, then add talcum powder and mix thoroughly.

(4) Insert capsule shell bodies (size 1) into the capsule plate (see Appendix ID for details), then place mixed powders on the capsule filling plate by gently tapping the capsule plate until the powders thoroughly filled in the capsule shell bodies, finally put capsule shell caps on.

3. Quick-acting cold capsule (plate filling)

1) Formulation:

Acetaminophen	300 g
Vitamin C	100 g
Bile powder	100 g
Caffeine	3 g
Chlorpheniramine	3 g
10% starch slurry	q. s.
Food colorant	q. s.
Obtain	1 000 capsules

2) Procedures:

(1) Grind the drugs, pass them through the 80-mesh sieve separately.

(2) Weigh about 10 g of starch and disperse it evenly in 100 mL of distilled water, and heat to gelatinize (at $80 \sim 85$ ℃) to obtain 10% of starch paste. After cooling, divide starch paste into three parts: A, B and C. Add a small amount of edible carmine to part A to prepare the red paste; add a small amount of edible orange (maximum dose is 1/10 000) to part B to prepare the yellow paste; add no pigment to part C to prepare the white paste.

(3) Divide acetaminophen into three parts: part one is thoroughly mixed with chlorpheniramine and then with the red paste; part two is thoroughly mixed with bile powder and vitamin C, then with the yellow paste; part three is thoroughly mixed with caffeine and then with the white paste. Above three parts are prepared as soft materials separately, and pass them through a 14-mesh nylon sieve to prepare wet granules, then dry wet granules at 70 ℃ to ensure the water content is lower than 3%.

(4) Mix three kinds of granules thoroughly until the mixture established an even color.

(5) Insert the capsule shell bodies into the capsule plate (see Appendix ID for details), then put the mixed granules on the capsule filling plate. Gently tap the capsule plate until all the granules evenly filled in the capsule shell bodies, put capsule shell caps on.

[Precautions]

(1) The quick-acting cold capsule is a compound preparation in which doses of each ingredient varies remarkably. To avoid uneven mixing due to significantly different doses or densities and probable segregation phenomenon during filling process, the present experiment adopts granulation strategy before filling. Granulation is favorable for capsule filling due to increased mixing uniformity and enhanced fluidity of the powder.

(2) Since three kinds of granules assume three colors before mixing, the uniformity of mixed granules can be judged simply by the uniformity of the color.

VI. Experiment results and discussion

Capsules are measured by appearance, water, weight variation, and disintegration test.

1. Appearance

Capsules should be clean and tidy, and have no bond, deformation, leakage, breaks and abnormal odor.

2. Water

Water determination for Chinese medicine hard capsules is required and should be conducted according to Determination of Water (0832, ChP 2020). Unless otherwise specified, the water content should be not more than 9.0%.

3. Weight variation

Unless otherwise specified, take 20 capsules (10 capsules for Chinese medicines), weigh accurately and separately. Open each capsule without loss of shell material, and remove the content as completely as possible. Clean the shell with a small brush or other appropriate tool. Weigh the shell of each capsule, calculate the weight of content and the average weight. Compare the content of each capsule with the average (capsules with labeled weight should be compared with the labeled weight). Not more than 2 capsules should deviate from the average (or labeled) weight by more than one weight variation limit shown in Table 3 – 23 and none should deviate by more than twice the limit. Fill the results in Table 3 – 24.

Table 3 – 23　Weight variation limit of capsules

Average or labeled weight	Weight variation limit
Less than 0.30 g	±10%
0.30 g or more	±7.5%

Table 3 –24 Results of weight variation test

Number	Capsule weight/g	Shell weight/g	Content weight/g	Number	Capsule weight/g	Shell weight/g	Content weight/g
1				11			
2				12			
3				13			
4				14			
5				15			
6				16			
7				17			
8				18			
9				19			
10				20			
Average weight/g							
Weight variation limit/g							
Qualified or not							

4. Disintegration test

Unless otherwise specified, take 6 capsule samples, and determine their disintegration time by using a disintegration apparatus. If the capsules float on the surface of the water, a disk may be used. All those hard capsules should disintegrate within 30 min. If one of them fails to disintegrate completely, repeat the test on 6 other capsules. All those 6 capsules should meet the requirement. For capsules required to take the drug dissolution or release test, the disintegration test is not required.

VII. Questions

(1) What roles do talcum powder and starch play in the formulation of analgesic capsule of corydalis tuber?

(2) What indicators can be used to evaluate the fluidity of powder?

实验七 片剂的制备及质量评价

一、实验目的

（1）掌握湿法制粒压片法的制备工艺。
（2）掌握片剂的质量检查方法。
（3）熟悉旋转压片机的结构和操作。

二、实验原理

片剂（tablets）系指原料药物或与适宜的辅料制成的片状制剂。片剂具有剂量准确、化学稳定性好、携带方便、生产成本低、制备的机械化程度高等特点，因此在现代药物制剂中应用最为广泛。

根据给药途径片剂可分为口服用片剂、口腔用片剂、外用片剂等。口服片剂又可分为普通片、包衣片、泡腾片、咀嚼片、分散片、缓释片、控释片、多层片等多种类型。

片剂的制备方法按制备工艺分为制粒压片法和直接压片法。制粒压片又分为湿法制粒压片和干法制粒压片。直接压片法又可分为直接粉末压片和空白颗粒压片法。

湿法制粒压片法工艺流程如图 3-10 所示。前半部分与湿法制备颗粒剂相同，即需要先加入适量润湿剂或黏合剂制软材，软材的干湿程度对片剂的质量影响较大，以"握

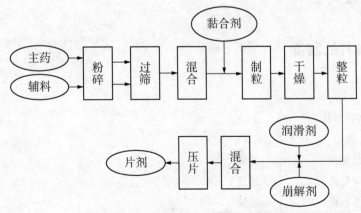

图 3-10 湿法制粒压片的工艺流程

之成团，轻压即散"为宜。湿颗粒干燥后，需过筛整粒以便将粘连的颗粒散开，随后加入润滑剂压片。

阿司匹林（乙酰水杨酸）是水杨酸的衍生物。作为一种非甾体抗炎药，阿司匹林常用于治疗发热、疼痛及类风湿关节炎等，其微溶于水，易溶于乙醇，遇水易水解，可生成对胃黏膜有强刺激性的水杨酸和醋酸。阿司匹林的常见剂型有片剂、胶囊、栓剂等。

片剂的质量检查项目包括性状、重量差异、含量测定、硬度、脆碎度、崩解时限和溶出度等。硬度是片剂的径向破碎力，是评价片剂质量最简便的方法，可用硬度测定仪测定。脆碎度可以评价非包衣片的脆碎情况和其他物理强度，如压碎强度等，可用脆碎度检查仪进行测定。

三、预习思考

（1）片剂常用的辅料有哪几大类？各举 2～3 个例子说明。

（2）阿司匹林的结构特点？根据阿司匹林的结构特点，在阿司匹林片的处方设计时辅料的选择应注意哪些问题？

（3）制备阿司匹林片的过程中，如何减少阿司匹林的水解？

四、实验材料与仪器

1. 实验试剂与试药

阿司匹林、淀粉、柠檬酸、滑石粉。

2. 实验仪器

旋转式多冲压片机、崩解仪、硬度计、脆碎度测定仪、恒温水浴锅、烘箱、尼龙筛网、烧杯、瓷盘等。

五、实验内容

阿司匹林片的制备

1. 处方

阿司匹林	30 g
淀粉	6.0 g
柠檬酸	适量
10% 淀粉浆	适量
滑石粉	适量
共制成	100 片

2. 实验步骤

（1）黏合剂的制备：将 0.2 g 枸橼酸溶于约 20 mL 蒸馏水中，加入淀粉约 2 g 分散均匀，加热糊化（80～85 ℃），得 10% 淀粉浆。

（2）湿颗粒的制备：阿司匹林粉碎过 100 目筛。取处方量的阿司匹林与淀粉混合均匀，加适量 10% 淀粉浆制软材，过 16 目筛制粒，将湿颗粒于 60 ℃ 干燥 1 h，过 16 目和 60 目筛整粒。干颗粒称重，加入相当于颗粒量 3% 的滑石粉，混匀。

（3）压片：将颗粒倾入压片机，调节片重约为 0.36 g 进行压片。旋转式多冲压片机使用说明见附录 IG。

注意事项

（1）淀粉浆制好后应稍加冷却后制粒，避免淀粉浆温度过高影响药物稳定性；温度也不宜过低，黏度大不易分散均匀。

（2）制粒后应立即干燥，干燥温度不宜超过 60 ℃。

（3）阿司匹林水解受金属离子催化，制粒时不宜选用金属筛而宜选择尼龙筛。

3. 质量检查

（1）重量差异：参照 2020 版《中国药典》通则 0101 片剂"重量差异"项进行测定。取供试品 20 片，精密称定总质量，求得平均片重后，再分别精密称定每片的质量，每片质量与平均片重比较，按表 3－25 中的规定，超出重量差异限度的不得多于 2 片，并不得有 1 片超出限度 1 倍。将测得的结果填入表 3－25。

表 3－25　重量差异限度

平均片重或标示片重	重量差异限度
0.3 g 以下	±7.5%
0.3 g 及以上	±5%

（2）硬度：取供试品 6 片，分别将其径向置于硬度仪两个柱杆之间，顺时针旋转手柄使柱杆对片剂径向加压，当片剂破碎时，仪器显示的压力即为片剂的硬度（单位为 N），随后逆时针旋转手柄，清除残留的碎片。测定 6 片的硬度，计算平均值。

（3）脆碎度：片重为 0.65 g 或以下者取若干片，使其总质量约为 6.5 g；片重大于 0.65 g 者取 10 片，用吹风机吹去脱落的粉末，精密称重，置脆碎度测定仪圆筒中，转动 100 次。取出，同法除去粉末，精密称重，减失质量不得超过 1%，且不得检出断裂、龟裂及粉碎的片。本试验一般仅做 1 次。当减失质量超过 1% 时，应复测 2 次，3 次的平均减失质量不得过 1%，并不得检出断裂、龟裂及粉碎的片。方法详见 2020 年版《中国药典》（通则 0923）片剂脆碎度检查法。

（4）崩解时限：除另有规定外，取供试品 6 片，分别置升降式崩解仪吊篮的玻璃管中（浸入 37 ℃ 的水中），启动崩解仪进行检查。崩解仪按一定频率和幅度往返运动。从片剂置于玻璃管时开始计时，至片剂破碎且全部固体粒子都通过玻璃管底部的筛网为止，记录片剂的崩解时间。片剂的崩解时限如表 3-26 所示。按规定，阿司匹林片应在 15 min 全部崩解。如有 1 片不能完全崩解，应另取 6 片复试，均应符合规定。方法详见 2020 年版《中国药典》（通则 0921）崩解时限检查法。崩解仪使用说明见附录 IE。

表 3-26　片剂的崩解时限

片剂	普通片	浸膏片	糖衣片	薄膜包衣片	肠溶包衣片
崩解时限/min	15	60	60	30	人工胃液中 2 h 不得有裂缝、崩解或软化；人工肠液中 60 min 内全部崩解

（5）考察润滑剂用量对片剂的硬度、崩解时限和重量差异的影响。保持处方其他条件不变，改变滑石粉用量，使滑石粉的量分别为颗粒质量的 1%、3%、4% 和 5%，比较 4 种片剂的硬度、崩解时限和重量差异。

六、实验结果与讨论

1. 片剂的外观性状、硬度和崩解时限

将测得的结果填入表 3-27。

表 3-27　片剂外观性状、硬度及崩解时限

编号	外观	硬度/N	崩解时限/min
1			
2			
3			
4			
5			
6			

2. 片剂的重量（简称片重）差异

将测得的结果填入表 3-28。

表 3-28　片重差异

编号	片重/mg	编号	片重/mg
1		11	
2		12	
3		13	
4		14	
5		15	
6		16	
7		17	
8		18	
9		19	

续表 3 - 28

编号	片重/mg	编号	片重/mg
10		20	

平均片重/g:

重量差异合格范围/g:

结论:

3. 片剂的脆碎度

将测得的结果填入表 3 - 29。

表 3 - 29 片剂脆碎度

片数	试验前重/g	试验后重/g	脆碎度/%

结论:

4. 润滑剂用量对片剂质量的影响

将测得的结果填入表 3 - 30、表 3 - 31。

表 3 - 30 滑石粉用量对片剂硬度的影响

滑石粉用量	硬度/N						
	1	2	3	4	5	6	平均
1%							
3%							
4%							
5%							

表 3 - 31 滑石粉用量对片剂崩解时限和重量差异的影响

滑石粉用量	崩解时间（6片）/min	硬度（6片）/N	片重差异（20片）/g
1%			
3%			
4%			
5%			

七、思考题

（1）处方中加入柠檬酸的目的是什么?

（2）为什么要用尼龙筛网制粒?

（3）阿司匹林片的润滑剂可以用硬脂酸镁替代滑石粉吗? 为什么?

（4）片剂重量差异不合格的主要原因是什么?

（5）简要说明片剂硬度和崩解时限不合格的主要原因和解决方法。

Experiment 7   Preparation and Quality Inspections of Aspirin Tablets

I. Purpose

(1) To master wet granulation process for preparation of tablets.

(2) To master quality control methods of tablets.

(3) To be familiar with construction and use of the rotary tablet machine.

II. Principles

Tablets are solid dosage forms prepared by compression of active substances with suitable excipients. Tablets are characterized by accurate dosage, high stability, portability, low cost, and high mechanization. Therefore, tablets are widely used in modern pharmaceutical preparations.

According to the route of administration, tablets are divided into oral tablets, tablets for use in the mouth, and tablets for external use. Oral tablets mainly include uncoated tablets, coated tablets, effervescent tablets, chewable tablets, dispersible tablets, sustained-release tablets, controlled-release tablets and multilayer tablets.

The preparation methods of tablets are broadly classified into direct compression and granulation tableting. Granulation tableting can be divided into dry granulation tableting and wet granulation tableting. Direct compression can be divided into direct powder compression and blank granulation compression.

The process of wet granulation tableting is illustrated in Figure 3 – 10. Wet granulation needs to make soft materials through adding wetting agents or adhesives. The humidity of soft materials has the critical effect on the quality of tablets. Soft materials are considered appropriate, when they can be gripped into clumps, pressed to spallation but not fragmented in pow-

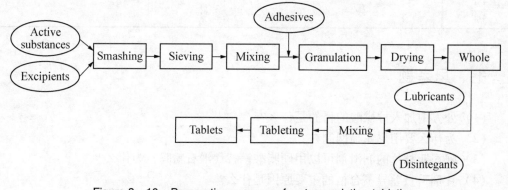

Figure 3 – 10   Preparation process of wet granulation tableting der. Press soft materials to pass through sieves to obtain wet granules. After drying, granules need to screen to disperse adhesive granules and then lubricants are added.

Aspirin (acetylsalicylic acid) is a salicylic acid derivative. As a non-steroidal anti-inflammatory drug, it is usually used to treat fever, pain, and rheumatoid arthritis, etc. Aspirin dissolves slightly in water but easily in ethanol. It is easy to hydrolyze in water, and produce salicylic acid and acetic acid, which strongly irritate to gastric mucosa. The common dosage forms of aspirin include tablets, capsules, and suppository, etc.

Quality inspections of tablets mainly include character, weight variation, contents, hardness, friability, disintegration, and dissolution. Hardness, representing radical crushing force of tablets, which can be determined by hardness tester, is the easiest way to evaluate the quality of tablets. Friability is used to evaluate the fragility and other physical strength of the uncoated tablets, such as crushing strength. It can be determined by friability test.

III. Preview

(1) What are the commonly used excipients in tablets? Please give 2 ~ 3 examples for each kind of excipients, respectively.

(2) What are the structural characteristics of aspirin? Based on these characteristics, what critical factors should be considered in choosing excipients for aspirin tablets.

(3) When preparing tablet, how to avoid the hydrolysis of aspirin?

IV. Experiment materials and equipments

1. Reagents and experimental materials

Aspirin, starch, citric acid and talcum powder.

2. Experimental equipments

Rotary multiple punch tablet machine, disintegration tester, hardness tester, friability tester, thermostat water bath, drying oven, nylon sieve, beaker and porcelain plate.

V. Experiment contents

Preparation of aspirin tablets

1) Formulation:

Aspirin	30 g
Starch	6.0 g
Citric acid	q. s.
10% Starch paste	q. s.
Talcum powder	q. s.
Obtain	100 tablets

2) Procedures:

(1) Preparation of adhesives. Add 0.2 g of citric acid into 20 mL of distilled water, and

then add 2 g of starch to mix and heat at $80 \sim 85$ ℃ for gelatinization to obtain 10% starch paste.

(2) Preparation of wet granules. Smash aspirin and screen through 100 mesh sieve. Mix aspirin and starch according to the formulation, and then add 10% starch paste to make soft materials. Pass through a 16 mesh sieve for granulation. Dry granules at 60 ℃ for 1 h, and then screen them by a 16 mesh sieve and 60 mesh sieve. Weigh dried granules and mix them with 3% talcum powder.

(3) Compression. Pour granules into a rotary tablet machine and adjust the mass of individual tablets to about 0.36 g. See Appendix ⅠG for instructions of rotary tablet machine.

[**Precautions**]

(1) Starch paste should cooled before granulation to avoid overheating and affecting drug stability.

(2) After granulation, granules should be dried immediately below 60 ℃.

(3) The hydrolysis of aspirin is catalyzed by metal ions, so it's appropriate to select nylon sieves for granulation rather than wire sieves.

3) Quality inspections：

(1) Weight variation. The determination refers to ChP 2020 0101 weight variation. Take 20 tablets and calculate the average weight, and then weigh individually and accurately. Compare the weight of each tablet with the average weight. According to the requirements stated in the Table 3 – 25, no more than 2 of the individual weights exceed the weight variation limit and none doubles the limits.

Table 3 –25   Weight variation limit

Average or labeled weight	Weight variation limit
Less than 0.3 g	±7.5%
0.3 g or more	±5%

(2) Hardness. Take 6 tablets and place them radially between the movable platens of the hardness tester, so that compression occurs across the diameter. The force required to cause tablets break is called hardness (N). Determine individually 6 tablets and calculate the average hardness.

(3) Friability. When tablets with a unit weight equal to or less than 0.65 g, take a sample of whole tablets corresponding as near as possible to 6.5 g. When tablets with a unit weight of more than 0.65 g, take a sample of 10 whole tablets. The tablets should be carefully dedusted prior to testing. Accurately weigh the tablet sample, and place the tablets in the drum of the friability tester. Rotate the drum 100 times, and remove the tablets. Remove dust from the tablets as before, and accurately weigh. The weight loss from the sample is not more than 1.0%, and

no cracked, cleaved, or broken tablets are present in the sample. The test should be repeated twice, if the weight lost is more than 1.0%. The average weight loss from three samples should not be more than 1.0%, and no cracked, cleaved, or broken tablets are present. More details are shown in rule 0923 friability test, ChP 2020.

(4) Disintegration. Unless specified otherwise, take 6 tablets and place 1 in each of the six tubes of the basket in disintegration tester (immerse in 37 ℃ water). Operate the apparatus to raise and lower the basket at a constant frequency and extent. Test begins when tablets are put in tubes, and the time that tablets disintegrate completely and all particles move through sieves under the bottom of tubes is the disintegration time of corresponding tablets. According to the requirements stated in the Table 3 – 26, all of the tablets should disintegrate within 15 min. If 1 tablet fails to disintegrate, repeat the test on 6 additional tablets. All the tablets should comply with the requirements. More details are shown in rule 0921 disintegration Test, ChP 2020. See Appendix ⅠE for instructions of disintegration tester.

Table 3 –26　Disintegration limit

Tablets	Common tablets	Extract tablets	Sugar coated tablets	Film coated tablets	Enteric coated tablets
Disintegration time limit/min	15	60	60	30	Tablets show no evidence of disintegration, cracking or softening in simulated gastric fluid within 2 h, but disintegrate completely in simulated intestinal fluid within 60 min

(5) Effects of the amount of talcum powder on hardness, disintegration and weight variation of tablets. Adjust the amount of talcum powder in the preparations to 1%, 3%, 4% and 5% of granule weight without changing other conditions. Compare the difference among these four kinds of tablets in hardness, disintegration and weight variation.

Ⅵ. Experiment results and discussion

(1) Appearance, hardness and disintegration of tablets.
Fill the results in Table 3 – 27.

Table 3 –27　Appearance, hardness and disintegration of tablets

Number	Appearance	Hardness/N	Disintegration time/min
1			
2			
3			
4			
5			
6			

（2）The weight variation of tablets.

Fill the results in Table 3 – 28.

Table 3 – 28　Weight variation

Number	Weight/mg	Number	Weight/mg
1		11	
2		12	
3		13	
4		14	
5		15	
6		16	
7		17	
8		18	
9		19	
10		20	

Average weight/g：

Qualified range of weight/g：

Conclusion：

（3）Friability of tablets.

Fill the results in Table 3 – 29.

Table 3 – 29　Friability of tablets

Tablets number	Weight before test/g	Weight after test/g	Friability/%

Conclusion：

（4）Effects of the of talcum powder on the quality of tablets.

Fill the results in Table 3 – 30 and Table 3 – 31.

Table 3 – 30　Effects of the amount of talcum powder on hardness

Talcum powder	Hardness/N						
	1	2	3	4	5	6	Average
1%							
3%							
4%							
5%							

Table 3 –31　Effects of the amount of talcum powder on disintegration and weight variation

Talcum powder	Disintegration time (6 tablets) /min	Hardness (6 tablets) /N	Weight variation (20 tablets)/g
1%			
3%			
4%			
5%			

VII. Questions

(1) What is the purpose of adding citric acid in the preparation of aspirin tablets?

(2) Why are nylon sieves chosen for granulation?

(3) Can magnesium stearate replace talcum powder in aspirin tablets?

(4) What are the main reasons for the unqualified weight variation?

(5) Please explain briefly the main reasons for the unqualified hardness and disintegration of tablets and give some solutions.

实验八　片剂的包衣

一、实验目的

(1) 掌握薄膜包衣的制备工艺和质量要求。

(2) 掌握肠溶包衣的制备工艺和质量要求。

(3) 熟悉影响包衣质量的主要因素。

二、实验原理

将包衣材料涂覆在片剂（素片或称片芯）表面，使其干燥后成为紧密被覆在片剂表面的一层或多层衣层的过程，称为片剂包衣（tablet coating）。根据包衣材料的不同，可将包衣分为包糖衣和包薄膜衣两大类别。包薄膜衣是目前最常用的包衣方法，系指在片芯表面涂覆高分子聚合物，片剂包薄膜衣后称为薄膜衣片。薄膜衣又可分为胃溶型、肠溶型和水不溶型（缓释型）。通常情况下，除非特别说明，"薄膜衣片"特指胃溶型薄膜衣片。

薄膜包衣通常被认为是增强片剂性能最经济的方法：①可优化产品外观；②改良产品的口味及气味；③使产品便于吞咽；④防潮/避光/隔绝空气，增加药物稳定性；⑤增强速释片剂的物理完整性；⑥包衣后可印字使产品易于识别；⑦肠溶型和不溶型包衣可控制药物释放部位及释放速度；⑧将有配伍禁忌的药物分别置于片芯和衣层制备复方片剂。另外，薄膜包衣具有成膜材料用量少，操作简便，对药物崩解和溶出的不良影响小等优点，因而在制剂生产中得到广泛应用。薄膜包衣的工艺流程如图 3 - 11 所示。包肠溶衣时，为减少片芯的吸潮或避免药物与肠衣层的相互作用，可在片芯和肠衣层之间加包隔离层。

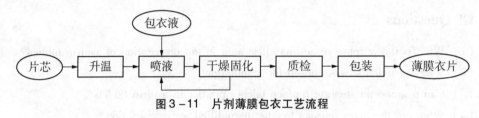

图 3 - 11　片剂薄膜包衣工艺流程

胃溶型、肠溶型和水不溶型薄膜衣通常采用不同的包衣材料来实现。常用的胃溶型包衣材料包括亲水性纤维素衍生物，以羟丙甲纤维素（hydroxypropyl methylcellulose，HPMC）应用最为广泛，商品化产品有欧巴代（Opadry）。另一种常用的胃溶型包衣材料是聚丙烯酸树脂类，如甲基丙烯酸二甲氨基乙酯 - 中性甲基丙烯酸酯共聚物，国产商品名为丙烯酸树脂Ⅳ号。肠溶型包衣材料则以尤特奇（Eudragit）最具有代表性，为甲基丙烯酸和甲基丙烯酸甲酯的共聚物。不溶型包衣材料有疏水性纤维衍生物，如乙基纤维素等。包衣成膜材料欧巴代和尤特奇的介绍，详见附录ⅡA。

为降低包衣材料的玻璃化转变温度，增加衣层的柔韧性，可加入增塑剂（plasticizer）。常用的增塑剂有柠檬酸三乙酯、癸二酸二丁酯和丙二醇。为避免水分散体包衣干燥过程中片芯的粘连，水分散体包衣液中可加入抗粘剂（anti-adherents），如滑石粉、单硬脂酸甘油酯等。包衣液在搅拌过程中会产生大量泡沫，泡沫会在膜面形成小斑点，加入几滴甲基硅油作为消泡剂（defoaming agents）可消除或减少泡沫，有利于包衣的致密性。

阿司匹林是迄今为止临床应用最广泛的解热镇痛药。阿司匹林对湿、热不稳定，对阿司匹林片进行薄膜包衣可增强其防潮效果从而增加稳定性。其次，阿司匹林对胃有刺激性，对阿司匹林片进行肠溶包衣可避免阿司匹林在胃内释放从而显著减小阿司匹林对胃的刺激。本实验将阿司匹林片分别包薄膜衣和肠溶衣，以达到提高稳定性和减小其胃刺激性的目的。

三、预习思考

（1）片剂包衣可达到哪些目的？

（2）包衣对片芯有什么质量要求？

（3）常用的肠溶衣材料有哪些？

（4）阿司匹林肠溶片的溶出实验应如何设计？

四、实验材料与仪器

1. 实验试剂与试药

阿司匹林素片、欧巴代® amb Ⅱ、欧巴代®Ⅱ03K、尤特奇® L30D-55（水分散体）、滑石粉、柠檬酸三乙酯、二氧化钛、羧甲基纤维素钠、聚乙二醇6000、柠檬黄、蒸馏水、盐酸溶液（9→1 000）、磷酸缓冲盐溶液（pH 为6.8）、饱和氯化钾溶液、饱和氯化钠溶液。

2. 实验仪器

高效包衣机、磁力搅拌器、高速分散均质机、崩解仪、硬度计、脆碎度仪、恒温恒湿试验箱、吹风机、玻璃棒、烧杯、搅拌子、筛网、干燥器。

五、实验内容

（一）阿司匹林薄膜衣片

1. 包衣液的配制

取欧巴代®amb Ⅱ薄膜包衣预混剂15 g，搅拌状态下缓慢加入60 g蒸馏水中，持续搅拌（磁力搅拌）45 min，使其分散均匀。在整个包衣过程中，保持轻微搅拌使包衣液分散均匀。

2. 实验步骤

（1）取阿司匹林素片400 g，吹去表面的细粉或颗粒，置包衣锅内，关闭密封门。

（2）开启高效包衣机，待设备自检后，点击按键进入包衣机"工艺员模式"，设置相关参数。

（3）开启主机、风机、加热（功率2 kW），待包衣锅内物料（素片）温度上升至设定区间，依次开启顶针气源、雾化气源和蠕动泵，直至包衣液经蠕动泵从喷枪喷出雾状液滴。

（4）时时观察包衣状态，待包衣片面色泽均匀，增重约3%，依次关闭蠕动泵、雾化气源和顶针气源。继续加热2 min，待片剂干燥后关闭加热。报警温度降至40 ℃以下后，关闭风机与主机，最后关闭电源。打开包衣锅，取出包衣片成品。高效包衣机简介详见附录ⅠH。

> 注意事项

（1）配制包衣液时，应防止气泡产生，包衣过程中应持续搅拌使分散均匀，防止产生沉淀。包衣液宜现配现用。

（2）阿司匹林素片应有较大的硬度，耐磨。包衣前吹去素片表面的细粉，保持片面光洁。

（3）包衣过程中，应注意物料温度和进风温度的控制。温度过高则干燥太快而成膜不均匀，温度太低则干燥太慢易造成粘连。

（4）喷液速度及包衣锅转速应适宜，喷液速度过快易出现成膜不均匀、磕片现象。

（5）包衣过程中可使用长柄药匙经正面舱门小口取样观察，取样时尽量不要打开密封门。

（6）包衣结束后应及时清洗喷枪系统，防止残余包衣液凝结堵塞系统中的管道。

（二）阿司匹林肠溶衣片

1. 包隔离层

（1）包衣液的配制。

取欧巴代®Ⅱ03K 15 g，搅拌下缓慢加入 60 g 蒸馏水中，持续搅拌（磁力搅拌）45 min，使其分散均匀。

（2）取阿司匹林素片按阿司匹林薄膜衣包衣流程包隔离层至增重约 3%。

2. 包肠溶衣

包衣液的配制。

（1）处方：

尤特奇® L30D-55	47 g
滑石粉	6.4 g
柠檬酸三乙酯	1.4 g
二氧化钛	1.75 g
羧甲基纤维素钠	0.55 g
聚乙二醇 6000	0.55 g
柠檬黄	0.65 g
水	25 g
共制成	100 g

（2）实验步骤：将羧甲基纤维素钠溶于 5 g 水中，聚乙二醇溶于 1 g 水中。将这两种溶液加入 19 g 水中，使总水量为 25 g。将滑石粉、二氧化钛和色素加到上述混合溶液中，用高速分散均质机匀化 30 min。将上述均质化的混悬液缓慢地倒入尤特奇® L30D-55 水分散体中，低速搅拌混匀后过 100 目筛得包衣液。保持包衣液轻微搅拌至包衣结束。

包衣程序按照上述阿司匹林薄膜包衣片的制备进行，肠溶包衣片增重约 9%。

注意事项

（1）肠溶衣包衣液配制好后过100目筛，包衣全过程应保持包衣液处于轻微搅拌状态使其均匀分散以防沉淀。

（2）随着包衣液体积减少，应调慢搅拌转速，避免泡沫产生。

（三）主机转速和蠕动泵转速对包衣质量的影响

（1）保持其他工艺参数不变，设置主机转速为10 r/min，比较蠕动泵转速为2 r/min和10 r/min对包衣质量（外观、片重差异）的影响。

（2）保持其他工艺参数不变，设置蠕动泵转速为2 r/min，比较主机转速为5 r/min和10 r/min对包衣质量（外观、片重差异）的影响。

（四）肠溶包衣增重对片剂崩解时限的影响

取已经完成隔离层包衣的片剂，保持工艺参数不变，对片剂进行肠溶包衣，考察不同包衣增重（7%和15%）对崩解时限的影响。

（五）与市售阿司匹林肠溶片比较

取自制阿司匹林肠溶片和市售肠溶片（与自制相同标示量），比较两者硬度、脆碎度、崩解时限和片重差异，并分析产生差异的原因。

（六）质量检查

1. 外观性状

应色泽均匀，光洁、无杂斑，无异物。

2. 重量差异

参照片剂重量差异检查法（2020版《中国药典》通则0101）测定。取供试品20片，精密称定总质量，求得平均片重后，再分别精密称定每片的质量。每片质量与平均片重相比（表3-32），超出重量差异限度的药片不得多于2片，并不得有1片超出限度1倍。

表3-32　重量差异限度规定

平均片重或标示片重	重量差异限度
0.3 g以下	±7.5%
0.3 g及以上	±5%

3. 硬度

取供试品6片，分别将其径向置于硬度仪两个活动柱杆之间，顺时针旋转手柄对片剂径向加压，当片剂破碎时，仪器显示的压力即为片剂的硬度（单位为N），随后逆时针旋转手柄，清除残留的碎片。测定 6 片的硬度，计算平均值。

4. 脆碎度

参照片剂脆碎度检查法（2020 版《中国药典》通则 0923）测定。

取片重为 0.65 g 或以下者若干片，使其总质量约为 6.50 g；片重大于 0.65 g 者取 10 片，用吹风机吹去脱落的粉末，精密称重，置圆筒中，转动 100 次，取出，同法除去粉末，精密称重，减失质量不得超过 1%，且不得检出断裂、龟裂及粉碎的片。本试验一般仅做 1 次。当减失质量超过 1% 时，应复测 2 次。3 次测量的平均减失质量不得过 1%，并不得检出断裂、龟裂及粉碎的片。

5. 崩解时限

参照崩解时限检查法 2020 版《中国药典》通则 0921 测定，方法详见附录 IE。

阿司匹林薄膜衣片在盐酸溶液（9→1 000）中检查，应在 30 min 内全部崩解。如有 1 片不能完全崩解，应另取 6 片复试，均应符合规定。

阿司匹林肠溶衣片先在盐酸溶液（9→1 000）中检查 2 h，每片均不得有裂缝、崩解或软化现象；然后将吊篮取出，用少量水洗涤后，每管加入挡板 1 块，再在磷酸盐缓冲液（pH 为 6.8）中进行检查，肠溶片 1 h 内应全部崩解。如有 1 片不能完全崩解，应另取 6 片复试，均应符合规定。

6. 耐湿耐水性实验

将素片和薄膜衣片置于相对湿度 90% ±5% 的环境下（底部盛有 KNO_3 饱和溶液的 25 ℃干燥器中）放置 10 天，以片剂增重为指标，检查耐湿耐水性。若吸湿增重 5% 以上，则在相对湿度 75% ±5% 环境下（底部盛有 NaCl 饱和溶液的 25 ℃干燥器中）同法进行实验。若吸湿增重 5% 以下，其他考察项目符合要求，则不再进行此项试验。

六、实验结果与讨论

（1）素片及包衣片的质量检查结果。

将测得的结果填入表 3 – 33 中。

表 3 – 33　包衣前后片剂质量检查结果

片剂类型		素片	薄膜衣片	肠溶片
外观				
硬度/N				
脆碎度/%				
崩解时限/min	盐酸溶液（9→1 000）			
	磷酸盐缓冲液（pH 为 6.8）	—	—	
重量差异（是否合格）				
吸湿增重/%				

（2）主机转速和蠕动泵转速对包衣质量的影响。

将测得的结果填入表 3 - 34 中。

表 3 - 34　主机转速和蠕动泵转速对包衣质量的影响

转速			外观	重量差异 (Mean ± SD)
蠕动泵转速/ (2 r·min⁻¹)	主机转速/ (r·min⁻¹)	5		
		10		
主机转速/ (10 r·min⁻¹)	蠕动泵转速/ (r·min⁻¹)	2		
		10		

（3）肠溶衣增重对片剂崩解时限的影响。

将测得的结果填入表 3 - 35 中。

表 3 - 35　肠溶衣增重对片剂崩解时限的影响

肠溶衣增重/%	盐酸溶液（9→1 000）	磷酸缓冲液（pH 为 6.8）
7		
15		

（4）与市售阿司匹林肠溶片的比较。

将测得的结果填入表 3 - 36 中。

表 3 - 36　自制阿司匹林肠溶片与市售肠溶片的质量对比

肠溶片		自制肠溶片	市售肠溶片
外观			
硬度/N			
脆碎度/%			
崩解时限/ min	盐酸溶液 （9→1 000）		
	磷酸盐缓冲液 （pH 为 6.8）		
重量差异（Mean ± SD）			

七、思考题

（1）简述欧巴代包衣材料的种类、性质及其应用范围。

（2）简述尤特奇包衣材料的种类、性质及其应用范围。

（3）包衣过程影响包衣质量的影响因素有哪些？

（4）包衣时哪些因素会导致片剂表面粗糙、衣膜脱落？请提出解决方法。

Experiment 8　Coating of Tablets

Ⅰ. Purpose

(1) To master preparation process and quality inspections of film-coated tablets.

(2) To master preparation process and quality inspections of enteric-coated tablets.

(3) To be familiar with main factors affecting the quality of films.

Ⅱ. Principles

Tablet coating means a process that tablets (plain tablets or cores) are coated with coating materials to form one or more tight layers adhering on the surface of tablets after drying. Depending on coating materials, coating is divided into two categories: sugar coating and film coating, and the latter is the most commonly used coating method in which polymers are applied. Tablets coated by film are called film-coated tablets, the film can be further divided into gastric-soluble, enteric-soluble, and water-insoluble film (delayed-release film). While in general, "film-coated tablets" in Chinese appearing in textbooks and papers refers to gastric-soluble film-coated tablets unless otherwise stated.

Film coating is considered to be the most economical strategy to promote the performance of tablets: ①beautifying appearance; ② masking unpleasant tastes and odors; ③ making tablets easy to swallow; ④ protecting ingredients from air, moisture or light to increase drug stability; ⑤ enhancing the physical integrity of fast-release tablets; ⑥ printing on the film for easy identification; ⑦controlling the site or rate of drug release by coating enteric or insoluble materials; ⑧ preparing compound tablets by loading incompatible drugs in the core and coating layers respectively. In addition, the advantages of film coating include only tiny amounts of materials needed, simple operation, and few negative effects on disintegration and dissolution. Thus, it is widely used in tablet coating. The process of film coating is shown in Figure 3 – 11. In the case of enteric coating, an isolating layer can be added between the core and the enteric layers in order to reduce moisture absorption of the core and to avoid the interaction between the drug and enteric layers.

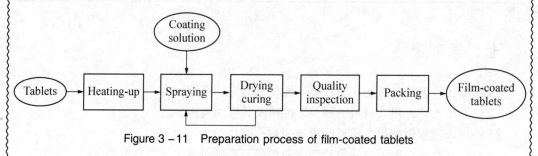

Figure 3 – 11　Preparation process of film-coated tablets

Different coating materials can be used to prepare different coated tablets such as gastric-soluble, enteric-soluble, and water-insoluble ones. Gastric-soluble coating materials include hydrophilic cellulose derivatives such as hydroxypropyl methylcellulose (HPMC), among which Opadry is widely used. Another commonly used gastric-soluble coating materials are polyacrylic resins such as dimethylaminoethyl methacrylate-neutral methacrylate copolymer whose domestic trade name is acrylic resin Ⅳ. The most representative enteric polymer is Eudragit, a copolymer with methacrylic acid and methyl methacrylate. The introduction to Opadry and Eudragit see Appendix ⅡA for details.

Plasticizers such as triethyl citrate, dibutyl sebacate and propylene glycol can attenuate glass transition temperature of coating materials and increase the plasticity and toughness of films. To avoid the adhesion of cores caused by drying during coating, anti-adherents such as talcum powder, glyceryl monostearate are frequently added to aqueous dispersion.

A few drops of methyl silicone oil are added as defoaming agents to eliminate or reduce a large amount of bubbles in coating solution under stirring, hence avoiding the formation of small spots on the surface of tablets. Moreover, defoaming facilitates to strengthen the compactness of films.

Aspirin is the most widely used antipyretic analgesic in clinical practice so far. Film coating to aspirin tablets can improve moisture-proof, thereby increase the stability of aspirin in terms of its instability to humidity and heat. Secondly, aspirin is irritant to stomach, which can be prevented by enteric coating due to avoiding the release of aspirin in stomach. In this experiment, aspirin film-coated tablets and enteric-coated tablets are prepared to improve their stability and reduce gastric irritation separately.

Ⅲ. Preview

(1) What objectives can be achieved by tablet coating?

(2) What are the quality requirements for cores of coated tablets?

(3) What kinds of enteric-coating materials are commonly used?

(4) Try to design dissolution test of aspirin enteric-coated tablets.

Ⅳ. Experiment materials and equipments

1. Reagents and experimental materials

Aspirin tablets, Opadry® amb Ⅱ, Opadry® Ⅱ03K, Eudragit® L30D-55 (aqueous dispersion), talcum powder, triethyl citrate, titanium dioxide, sodium carboxymethyl cellulose, PEG 6000, lemon yellow, distilled water, hydrochloric acid solution (HCl, 9→1 000), phosphate buffer solution (PBS, pH = 6.8), saturated solution of potassium nitrate (KNO_3), saturated solution of sodium chloride (NaCl).

2. Experimental equipments

High-efficiency coating machine, magnetic stirrer, high speed dispersion homogenizer, disintegration tester, hardness tester, friability tester, constant temperature and humidity test chamber, blower, glass rod, beaker, stirrer, sieve, desiccator.

V. Experiment contents

1. Preparation of aspirin film-coated tablets.

1) Preparation of coating solution. Slowly add 15 g of Opadry® amb Ⅱ coating premixture into 60 g of distilled water under stirring, stir continuously for 45 min to obtain coating solution. Keep coating solution uniformly dispersed by a slight agitation throughout the coating process.

2) Experimental procedures.

(1) Take 400 g of aspirin plain tablets, dedust powders or particles on the surface of tablets. Place them into the coating pan and then close the sealed door.

(2) Operate high-efficiency coating machine. After self-checking, press the button to enter the "crafter mode" and set up relevant parameters.

(3) Turn on the mainframe, fan and heater (power is 2 kW). When the temperature of materials (plain tablets) in pan reach setting value, turn on the air ejector pin, nebulizer and peristaltic pump in turn to let coating solution spray constantly from the spray gun in the form of fog droplets.

(4) Observe the coating process frequently until the color of tablets is uniform and the weight gain is about 3%. Turn off the peristaltic pump, nebulizer and air ejector pin in turn, and continually heat for 2 min to dry tablets, then turn off the heater. When alarm temperature drops below 40 ℃, turn off the fan, mainframe, and power. Open the coating pan and remove tablets. The introduction to high-efficiency coating machine see Appendix ⅠH for details.

[Precautions]

(1) When preparing coating solution, avoid the generation of bubbles as possible. Keep uniform dispersion of coating solution by slight agitating to avoid precipitation during the coating process. The coating solution is prepared just before use.

(2) Aspirin plain tablets must be hard and wearable. Dedust superficial powders or particles to keep the surface of tablets smooth prior to coating.

(3) Pay more attention to the temperature of materials and inlet air during coating procedure. Too high temperature, accompanied by rapid drying, will result in uneven film. While too lower temperature will cause adhesion due to slow drying.

(4) The speeds of spray and rotation should be matched. Too fast speed will cause uneven film or make tablets out-of-flatness.

(5) Use a long handle spoon to take samples through the small window of the front door during coating, avoid frequently opening the sealed door.

(6) When coating finishes, the spray gun system should be cleaned in time to prevent the

residual from clogging and blocking the pipeline of the system.

2. Preparation of aspirin enteric-coated tablets

1) Coating isolation layer.

(1) Preparation of coating solution.

Add slowly 15 g of Opadry® II 03K into 60 g of distilled water under agitation. Then continuously stir for 45 min to mix well.

(2) Coat isolation layer as described above to obtain weight gain about 3%.

2) Coating enteric layer.

Preparation of coating solution.

A. Formulation:

Eudragit® L30D-55	47 g
Talcum powder	6.4 g
Triethyl citrate	1.4 g
Titanium dioxide	1.75 g
Sodium carboxymethyl cellulose	0.55 g
PEG6000	0.55 g
Lemon yellow	0.65 g
Distilled water	25 g
Obtain	100 g

B. Preparation:

Dissolve sodium carboxymethyl cellulose and polyethylene glycol in 5 g and 1 g of distilled water, respectively. Then put them into 19 g of distilled water totally. Add talcum powder, titanium dioxide and lemon yellow to the above mixed solution, homogenize for 30 min by high speed dispersion homogenizer. Pour the suspension into Eudragit® L30D-55 aqueous dispersion slowly and mix at a low speed. Pass the above mixture through 100-mesh sieve. Take the filtrate and maintain a uniform dispersion throughout coating by a slight agitation.

Coatings proceed as directed by aspirin film-coated tablets and the weight gain of enteric-coated tablets is about 9%.

[Precautions]

(1) Pass enteric coating solution through a 100-mesh sieve after preparation. Throughout the coating process, keep a slight stirring so that the coating suspension is evenly dispersed to prevent precipitation.

(2) As the volume of coating solution decreases, the agitation speed should be reduced to avoid foaming.

3. Effects of the rotation speeds of pan and peristaltic pump on the quality of coating

(1) Keep other parameters fixed, set the speed of pan rotation at 10 r/min, then compare

the effects of peristaltic pump rotation at 2 and 10 r/min on the quality of coating (appearance, weight variation).

(2) Keep other parameters fixed, set the speed of peristaltic pump rotation at 2 r/min, compare the effects of pan rotation at 5 and 10 r/min on the quality of coating (appearance, weight variation).

4. Effects of weight gain after enteric coating on the disintegration of tablets

Keep other parameters fixed, coat tablets by the enteric coating suspension and evaluate the effects of weight gain of 7% and 15% on the disintegration of tablets.

5. Comparison with the commercially available aspirin enteric-coated tablet

Take homemade aspirin enteric-coated tablets and commercially available enteric-coated tablets (with same labelled amount) and compare their hardness, friability, disintegration and weight variation, then analyze the reasons of difference.

6. Quality inspections

1) Appearance:

The tablets should be uniform in color, smooth, no speckle, no foreign matter.

2) Weight variation:

The determination of weight variation should comply with the Weight Variation Test of tablets (0101, ChP 2020). Take 20 tablets and calculate the average weight, and then weigh individually and accurately. Compare the weight of each tablet with the average weight. According to the requirements stated in Table 3 – 32, no more than 2 of individual weights exceed the weight variation limit and none doubles the limits.

Table 3 – 32   Weight variation limit

Average or labeled weight	Weight variation limit
Less than 0.3 g	±7.5%
0.3 g or more	±5%

3) Hardness:

Take 6 tablets and place them radially between the movable platens of hardness tester, so that compression occurs across the diameter. The force required to cause tablets break is called hardness (in N). Determine individually 6 tablets and calculate the average hardness.

4) Friability:

The determination of friability should comply with the Friability Test (0923, ChP 2020). When tablets with a unit weight equal to or less than 0.65 g, take a sample of whole tablets corresponding as near as possible to 6.50 g. When tablets with a unit weight of more than 0.65 g, take a sample of 10 tablets. Tablets should be carefully dedusted prior to testing. Accurately weigh tablets and place them in the drum of the friability tester. Rotate the drum 100 times and remove the tablets. Remove dust from the tablets as before, and accurately weigh. Generally, the weight loss from the sample is not more than 1.0%, and no cracked, cleaved, or broken tablets are present in the sample. The test should be repeated twice, if the weight lost is more than 1.0%. The average weight loss from three samples should not be more than 1.0%, and no cracked, cleaved, or broken tablets are present.

5) Disintegration:

The determination of disintegration should comply with the Disintegration Test (0921, ChP 2020). See Appendix ⅠE for details.

(1) Take 6 aspirin film-coated tablets and place them in disintegration tester containing HCl (9→1 000). All the tablets should disintegrate within 30 min. If 1 tablet fails to disintegrate, repeat the test on additional 6 tablets. All the tablets should comply with the requirements.

(2) Take 6 aspirin enteric-coated tablets and place them in disintegration tester containing HCl (9→1 000). All the tablets should show no evidence of cracking, disintegrating or softening in 2 hours. Remove the basket and wash with a small quantity of water. Add a disk to each tube, then place them in disintegration tester containing PBS solution (pH = 6.8). All tablets should disintegrate completely within 1 h. If 1 tablet fails to comply with the test, repeat the test on additional 6 tablets. All the tablets should comply with the requirements.

6) Moisture and water resistance test:

Place aspirin tablets and aspirin film-coated tablets in a desiccator with relative humidity of 90% ±5% (saturated solution of KNO_3) at 25 ℃ for 10 days. The weight gain is used as an indicator to evaluate the moisture-resistance of tablets. If weight gain is more than 5%, place tablets in a desiccator with relative humidity of 75% ±5% (saturated solution of NaCl). If weight gain is less than 5% and other quality inspections meet the requirements, the test will not be conducted.

Ⅵ. Experiment results and discussion

1. Quality inspections of aspirin tablets and aspirin coated tablets

Fill the result in Table 3 – 33.

Table 3 – 33　Quality inspections of aspirin tablets before and after coating

Type of tablets		Plain tablets	Film-coated tablets	Enteric-coated tablets
Appearance				
Hardness/N				
Friability/%				
Disintegration limit time/min	HCl (9→1 000)			
	PBS (pH = 6.8)	—	—	
Weight variation (whether qualified)				
Moisture weight gain/%				

2. Effects of the rotation speeds of pan and peristaltic pump on the quality of coating

Fill the result in Table 3 – 34.

Table 3 – 34   Effects of the rotation speeds of pan and peristaltic pump on quality of coating

Rotation speed			Appearance	Weight variation ($Mean \pm SD$)
Peristaltic pump (2 r $\cdot$ min^{-1})	Pan/ (r $\cdot$ min^{-1})	5		
		10		
Pan/ (10 r $\cdot$ min^{-1})	Peristaltic pump (r $\cdot$ min^{-1})	2		
		10		

3. Effects of the weight gain after enteric coating on the disintegration of tablets

Fill the result in Table 3 – 35.

Table 3 – 35   Effects of the weight gain after enteric coating on the disintegration of tablets

Weight gain/%	HCl ($9 \rightarrow 1\ 000$)	PBS ($pH = 6.8$)
7		
15		

4. Comparison with commercially available aspirin enteric-coated tablets

Fill the result in Table 3 – 36.

Table 3 – 36   Comparison the homemade with commercially available aspirin enteric-coated tablets

Enteric-coated tablet		Homemade tablets	Commercially available tablets
Appearance			
Hardness/N			
Friability/%			
Disintegration time limit/min	HCl ($9 \rightarrow 1\ 000$)		
	PBS ($pH = 6.8$)		
Weight variation ($Mean \pm SD$)			

VII. Questions

(1) Briefly describe the types, characteristics and application of Opadry coating materials in pharmaceutical industry.

(2) Briefly describe the types, characteristics and application of Eudragit coating materials in pharmaceutical industry.

(3) What are the factors that greatly influence the quality of coated tablets during coating?

(4) What kinds of reasons would result in a rough surface of tablets or films falling-off during coating? Please give some solutions.

实验九　片剂溶出度的测定

一、实验目的

（1）掌握片剂溶出度的测定方法。

（2）熟悉溶出试验设计需要考虑的因素。

（3）熟悉溶出试验仪的结构及操作注意事项。

二、实验原理

片剂或胶囊等固体制剂口服后，在胃肠道中须经过崩解和溶出两个过程，其中的药物才能被吸收。对于高渗透性的药物来说，其口服吸收的程度通常与药物从固体制剂中溶出的速度与程度相关。我们通常将在指定的介质中，在一定的试验条件下，药物从片剂或胶囊等固体制剂溶出的速度和程度称为溶出度（dissolution）。在实际应用中，溶出度常用一定时间内药物的溶出百分率表示。难溶性药物的口服固体制剂均应做溶出度检查。《中国药典》和许多其他国家药典对口服固体制剂的溶出度及其测定方法都有明确规定。2020 版《中国药典》收载的溶出度测定法有转篮法、浆法、小杯法、桨碟法、转筒法、流通池法和往复筒法。溶出速度（dissolution rate）则指在单位时间内药物溶解的量，即溶出的速度。要加快机体对难溶性药物的吸收，不仅要增加药物溶出的程度，控制药物溶出的速度也非常重要。

溶出度试验在反映口服固体制剂内在品质方面发挥着重要作用。体外溶出试验的优劣以是否能反映制剂的内在品质为评判指标。对于创新药来说，适合的溶出方法可以使体外溶出曲线和体内吸收具有良好的相关性。对于仿制药物来说，溶出方法必须有足够的区分效应（体现制剂溶出情况的差异）。因要求自制制剂和原研药具有相似的溶出曲线，故须在不同溶出条件如水和多种 pH 的溶出介质（常用的有 pH = 1.2、pH = 4.0、pH = 6.8）中进行各制剂溶出曲线的测定和比对。溶出曲线相似性比较方法可见附录ⅢD。溶出介质的使用一般根据药物的性质和临床使用情况而定，可在溶出介质中添加表面活性剂，但应对添加种类和浓度进行评价。

除此之外，是选用浆法还是转篮法，装置是否加网碟，选择多大的转速等，都会对溶出方法的区分效应产生巨大的影响。应特别关注转速、溶出介质 pH 对溶出结果的影响。转速模拟的是胃肠道蠕动对药物溶出的影响，不同 pH 溶出介质则是反映药物在消化道不同部位的溶出情况。通常老年人的胃肠蠕动和胃酸分泌随年龄增长而急剧下降，若药物能在慢转速（50 r/min）条件和不同溶出介质中大部分溶出，则表明该制剂在胃肠蠕动较慢、胃酸分泌降低的老年人体内也可获得较高的生物利用度。

溶出度试验通常取 6 片（粒）进行，是否符合规定，有非常细化的判定标准，而不是简单的"均应超过限度"（具体判定标准见实验结果，应遵照执行）。凡检查溶出度或释放度的制剂，可不再进行崩解时限的检查。

三、预习思考

（1）2020 年版《中国药典》溶出度检查法有哪几种，各有什么适用范围？
（2）什么样的固体制剂需要进行溶出度检查？
（3）肠溶制剂的溶出介质有何要求？

四、实验材料与仪器

1. 实验试剂与试药

阿司匹林对照品、阿司匹林片、阿司匹林薄膜包衣片、阿司匹林肠溶片、盐酸、磷酸钠、氢氧化钠。

2. 实验仪器

溶出试验仪、紫外 - 可见分光光度计、天平、5 mL 注射器、0.45 μm 微孔滤膜、容量瓶。

五、实验内容

1. 溶出介质的配制

取稀盐酸 16.4 mL，加水稀释至 1 000 mL 配制酸性溶出介质（溶出介质 A）。

取溶出介质 A 750 mL，加入 0.2 mol/L 磷酸钠溶液 250 mL，用 2 mol/L 盐酸溶液或 2 mol/L 氢氧化钠溶液调节 pH 至 6.8，得磷酸盐缓冲液溶出介质（溶出介质 B，仅供肠溶片使用）。

2. 阿司匹林对照溶液的配制

精密称定阿司匹林对照品约 4 mg，用溶出介质 A 溶解并稀释至 100 mL，得浓度约为 40 μg/mL 的对照溶液 A。

精密称定阿司匹林对照品约 20 mg，用溶出介质 B 溶解并稀释至 100 mL，得浓度约为 200 μg/ml 的对照溶液 B（仅供肠溶片使用）。

3. 阿司匹林片和阿司匹林薄膜包衣片溶出度的测定

（1）预先用标准片对溶出试验仪进行校正。

（2）测定前用定位球调节桨叶底部距溶出杯的内底部为（25 ± 2）mm。分别量取经脱气处理的溶出介质 A 900 mL，置于各溶出杯内，实际量取的体积与规定体积偏差

应不超过 ±1%。

（3）待溶出介质温度恒定在（37 ± 0.5）℃，取供试品 6 片，分别投入溶出杯内，设定转速为 100 r/min，开启溶出试验仪。于 30 min 吸取溶出液约 10 mL，立即用 0.45 μm 的微孔滤膜滤过（取样至滤过应在 30 s 内完成）。

（4）取续滤液作为样品溶液，适当稀释后测定对照溶液 A 以及样品溶液在 276 nm 处的吸收度，计算阿司匹林片的溶出量和溶出百分率。

4. 阿司匹林肠溶片溶出度的测定

（1）将肠溶片投入预热至（37 ± 0.5）℃的 750 mL 的溶出介质 A 中，设定转速为 100 r/min，溶出 2 h 后取样 10 mL 滤过，补充相同体积的新鲜溶出介质 A。样品测定方法同上，计算药物在溶出介质 A 中的溶出量和溶出百分率。

（2）向上述溶出介质 A 中小心加入 37 ℃ 预热的 0.2 mol/L 磷酸钠溶液 250 mL，搅拌均匀，必要时用 2 mol/L 盐酸溶液或 2 mol/L 氢氧化钠溶液调节 pH 至 6.8，继续溶出 45 min，取样 10 mL，照上述测定方法，测定并计算阿司匹林肠溶片在溶出介质 B 中的溶出量和溶出百分率。

溶出试验仪使用说明详见附录 IH。

注意事项

（1）溶出介质使用前需新鲜配制并脱气。

（2）取样点应在桨叶上端距液面中间部位，离杯壁 10 mm。

（3）溶出介质加入后须盖上溶出杯的盖子，溶出介质无须过早预热，以免挥发致体积减小。

（4）片剂投入溶出杯后注意表面不应有气泡。

六、实验结果与讨论

1）计算药物的溶出百分率，判断溶出是否符合规定。

将测得的结果填入表 3 – 37 中。

表 3 –37　阿司匹林片的溶出度

编号	1	2	3	4	5	6	平均溶出度
溶出量/mg 溶出百分率/%							

≤Q　片　　　　≤Q – 10%　　片　　　　≤Q – 20%　　片

是否合格：

2）阿司匹林片（或薄膜包衣片）限度要求（Q）：30 min 溶出量应大于标示量

的 80%。

符合下述条件之一者，可判为符合规定：

（1）6 片中，每片的溶出量按标示量计算，均不低于规定限度（Q）；

（2）6 片中，如有 1～2 片低于 Q，但不低于 Q-10%，且其平均溶出量不低于 Q；

（3）6 片中，有 1～2 片低于 Q，其中仅有 1 片低于 Q-10%，但不低于 Q-20%，且其平均溶出量不低于 Q，应另取 6 片复试；初、复试的 12 片中有 1～3 片低于 Q，其中仅有 1 片低于 Q-10%，但不低于 Q-20%，且其平均溶出量不低于 Q。

以上结果判断中所示的 10% 和 20% 系指相对于标示量的百分率。

3）阿司匹林肠溶片限度要求（Q）：在溶出介质 A 中 2 h 的溶出量应小于标示量的 10%，随后置于溶出介质 B 中 45 min 溶出量应大于标示量的 70%。

符合下述条件之一者，可判为符合规定：

（1）溶出介质 A 中溶出量：

A. 6 片中，每片的溶出量均不大于 Q。

B. 6 片中，有 1～2 片大于 Q，但其平均溶出量不大于 Q。

（2）溶出介质 B 中溶出量：

A. 6 片中，每片的溶出量按标示量计算，均不低于 Q。

B. 6 片中，如有 1～2 片低于 Q，但不低于 Q-10%，且其平均溶出量不低于 Q。

C. 6 片中，有 1～2 片低于 Q，其中仅有 1 片低于 Q-10%，但不低于 Q-20%，且其平均溶出量不低于 Q，应另取 6 片复试；初、复试的 12 片中有 1～3 片低于 Q，其中仅有 1 片低于 Q-10%，但不低于 Q-20%，且其平均溶出量不低于 Q。

七、思考题

（1）试分析影响药物溶出度测定的因素。

（2）片剂的崩解时限合格，是否其溶出度一定合格，为什么？

（3）溶出度试验是否能反映固体制剂的内在品质，其判断标准是什么？

Experiment 9　Dissolution Test of Aspirin Tablets

Ⅰ. Purpose

（1）To master the operation of dissolution test.

（2）To be familiar with what should be considered before dissolution test.

（3）To be familiar with the structure of dissolution apparatus and its operating precautions.

Ⅱ. Principles

Solid dosage forms such as tablets and capsules disintegrate and dissolve in gastrointestinal tract prior to drug absorption. For drugs with high permeability, their oral absorption is related intensively to dissolution, which is defined as the rate and degree of drug dissolving from solid dosage forms in the specified media under certain conditions. In practical applications, dissolution is often expressed as the dissolution percentage of drugs within specified time interval. For poorly-soluble drugs, it is prerequisite to determine dissolution of their oral solid dosage forms. Pharmacopoeias of various countries set forth dissolution of oral solid dosage forms and their determination methods. The determination methods of dissolution in ChP 2020 include basket method, paddle method, small vessel method, paddle over disk method, rotating cylinder method, flow-through cell method and reciprocating cylinder method. Dissolution rate is defined as the amount of drugs dissolve per unit of time, that is, the speed of dissolution. Not only increasing the degree of dissolution, but also controlling dissolution rate is critical to promote the absorption of poorly-soluble drugs.

The dissolution test plays a critical role in reflecting the inherent qualities of oral solid dosage forms and whether it can reflect the inherent quality is the gold standard to judge the method good or not. For innovative drugs, an appropriate method contributes to a good correlation between *in vitro* dissolution and *in vivo* absorption. For generic drugs, the dissolution method must possess differentiating effect (exhibiting difference in dissolution of various preparations). Since generic drugs are required to possess the similar dissolution curve with reference listed drugs (RLD), the dissolution of samples should be tested under different dissolving conditions such as water and buffers with various pH (commonly pH = 1.2, 4.0 and 6.8). See Appendix ⅢD for details about comparison of similarity of dissolution curve. Screening dissolution medium is usually based on the properties of drugs and clinical application. Surfactants are allowed to add to media but before that, the types and concentrations of surfactants should be assessed.

Besides, choosing paddle method or basket method, adding disk or not, and different rotation rates of paddle or basket can remarkably affect the differentiating effect of dissolution. More attention should be paid to the rotation rates of paddle or basket and pH of media. The rotation rate simulates gastrointestinal peristalsis which greatly affects drug dissolution while pH of media reflects dissolving situation in the different parts of the digestive tract. In general, for elderly people, their gastrointestinal peristalsis and gastric acid secretion descend sharply with age. Therefore, if drugs can dissolve mostly in medium with different pH at a low rate (50 r/min), indicating that this preparation may possess good oral bioavailability in the elderly people who have sluggish gastrointestinal peristalsis and less gastric acid secretion.

The dissolution test is usually carried out using 6 tablets (capsules). Whether the dissolution complies with the regulations is not judged simply by "all require to exceed the limit". Instead, it is decided according to the detailed requirements stated in Experiment results part. For the preparations which are tested for dissolution or release, disintegration test is unnecessary.

Ⅲ. Preview

(1) How many dissolution methods are included in ChP 2020 and how about their appli-

cation?

(2) What kinds of solid dosage forms need dissolution test?

(3) What are the requirements for the dissolution media of enteric preparations?

IV. Experiment materials and equipments

1. Reagents and experimental materials

Reference standards of aspirin, aspirin tablets, aspirin thin film-coated tablets, aspirin enteric-coated tablets, hydrochloric acid, sodium phosphate and sodium hydroxide.

2. Experimental equipments

Dissolutionapparatus, UV-Vis spectrophotometer, balance, 5 mL syringe, 0. 45 μm microporous filter and volumetric flask.

V. Experiment contents

1. Preparation of dissolution medium

Take 16. 4 mL of hydrochloric acid and dilute it to 1 000 mL with distilled water, obtain acid dissolution medium (dissolution medium A).

Add 250 mL of 0. 2 mol/L tribasic sodium phosphate solution to 750 mL of dissolution medium A. Adjust pH to 6. 8, if necessary, with 2 mol/L hydrochloric acid or 2 mol/L sodium hydroxide, obtain phosphate buffer dissolution medium (dissolution medium B, only for enteric-coated tablets).

2. Preparation of aspirin standard solution

Weigh accurately reference substance of aspirin about 4 mg, dissolve and dilute with dissolution medium A, obtain 40 μg/mL standard solution A.

Weigh accurately reference substance of aspirin about 20 mg, dissolve and dilute with dissolution medium B, obtain 200 μg/mL standard solution B (only for enteric-coated tablets).

3. Dissolution tests for aspirin tablets and aspirin film-coated tablets

(1) Apply reference tablets for the calibration of dissolution apparatus.

(2) Before test, adjust the apparatus with positioning balls, making the distance between the inside bottom of the vessel and the bottom of the paddle blade is (25 ±2) mm. Add 900 mL of degassed dissolution medium A in each vessel. The deviation between the actual measured and the specified volume does not exceed ±1%.

(3) Maintain the temperature of dissolution medium at (37 ±0. 5) ℃, then place 1 tablet in each vessel (totally 6 vessels). Operate the apparatus at 100 r/min and timing starts. Withdraw 10 mL of medium at 30 min after adding tablets and filter it through 0. 45 μm microporous membrane immediately (sampling and filtering must be finished within 30 s).

(4) Take the filtrate as the sample solution, determine UV absorbances of standard solution A and the sample solution after dilution at 276 nm, calculate the amount and percentage of aspirin dissolved from tablets.

4. Dissolution test for aspirin enteric-coated tablets

(1) Adjust the apparatus and place enteric-coated tablets in 750 mL of dissolution medium A [pre-equilibrated to (37 ± 0.5) ℃]. Operate the apparatus at 100 r/min. After 2 h, withdraw 10 mL of medium and replace with equal volume of fresh dissolution medium A. Proceed according to the above method and calculated the amount and percentage of aspirin dissolved in dissolution medium A.

(2) Add 250 mL of 0.20 mol/L tribasic sodium phosphate [pre-heated to (37 ± 0.5) ℃] to each vessel containing 750 mL of dissolution medium A and 1 tablet. Adjust pH to 6.8 with 2 mol/L hydrochloric acid or 2 mol/L sodium hydroxide if necessary and continue to operate the apparatus for 45 min. Then withdraw 10 mL of medium and determine the content of aspirin as before, calculate the amount and percentage of aspirin dissolved in dissolution medium B.

See Appendix ⅠH for instructions of dissolution apparatus.

[**Precautions**]

(1) The dissolution medium should be freshly prepared and degassed before use.

(2) Sample between the surface of dissolution medium and the top of the blade, 10 mm away from the lateral vessel wall.

(3) Cover the vessels and preheat dissolution medium just before use to avoid the reduction of medium caused by volatilization.

(4) Exclude air bubbles on the surface of tablets.

Ⅵ. Experiment results and discussion

1) Calculate dissolution percentages of tablets at specified time. Evaluate whether dissolution meets the requirements. Fill the result in Table 3 – 37.

Table 3 – 37　Dissolution of aspirin tablets

Number	1	2	3	4	5	6	Average dissolution
The amount of drug dissolved/mg							
Dissolution percentage/%							

≤Q　　tablets	≤Q – 10%　　tablets	≤Q – 20%　　tablets
whether meet the requirements		

2) The requirement for aspirin tablets (or film-coated tablets) (Q): Not less than 80% of the labeled content dissolved within 30 min.

The requirement is met if the dissolution conforms to one of the following states.

（1）The amount of drug dissolved from each of 6 tablets is not below Q, calculated based on labeled content.

（2）If 1～2 of 6 tablets are below Q, but not less than Q－10% and the average amount of drug dissolved is not less than Q.

（3）If 1～2 of 6 tablets are below Q, only 1 tablet is less than Q－10%, but not less than Q－20%, and the average amount of drug dissolved is not less than Q, repeat the test on 6 additional tablets; if 1～3 of total 12 tablets are less than Q, and only 1 tablet is less than Q－10%, but not less than Q－20%, and the average amount of drug dissolved is not less than Q.

The 10% and 20% stated above are expressed as percentages of the labeled content.

3）The requirements for aspirin enteric-coated tablets（Q）: Not more than 10% of the labeled content dissolved in dissolution medium A within 2 h. Not less than 70% of the labeled content dissolved in dissolution medium B within 45 min.

The requirement is met if the dissolution conforms to one of the following states:

（1）The amount of drug dissolved in dissolution medium A:

A. The amount of drug dissolved from each of 6 tablets is not more than Q, calculated based on the labeled content.

B. If 1～2 of 6 tablets are more than Q, but the average amount of drug dissolved is not more than Q.

（2）The amount of drug dissolved in dissolution medium B:

A. The amount of drug dissolved from each of 6 tablets is not less than Q.

B. If 1～2 of 6 tablets are less than Q, but not less than Q－10% and the average amount of drug dissolved is not less than Q.

C. If 1～2 of 6 tablets are less than Q, only 1 tablet is less than Q－10%, but not less than Q－20%, and the average amount of drug dissolved is not less than Q, repeat the test on 6 additional tablets; if 1～3 of total 12 tablets are less than Q, and only 1 tablet is less than Q－10%, but not less than Q－20%, and the average amount of drug dissolved is not less than Q.

VII. Questions

（1）Analyze the factors that affect the determination of drug dissolution.

（2）If tablets comply with disintegration test, are they meet the requirements for dissolution?

（3）Can dissolution test reflect the inherent qualities of tablets, how to judge it?

实验十 软膏剂的制备

一、实验目的

（1）掌握不同类型软膏基质的处方与制备工艺。
（2）熟悉软膏中药物释放的测定方法及基质对药物释放的影响。

二、实验原理

软膏剂（ointments）系指原料药物与油脂性或水溶性基质混合制成的均匀半固体外用制剂。它可在应用部位发挥疗效或起保护和润滑皮肤的作用，药物也可吸收进入体循环产生全身治疗作用。根据原料药物在基质中分散状态不同，分为溶液型软膏剂和混悬型软膏剂。溶液型软膏剂为原料药物溶解（或共熔）于基质或基质组分中制成的软膏剂；混悬型软膏剂为原料药物细粉均匀分散于基质中制成的软膏剂。乳膏剂（creams）系指原料药物溶解或分散于乳状液型基质中形成的均匀半固体制剂。

基质（bases）是软膏剂及乳膏剂的赋形剂，它使软膏剂具有一定的剂型特性且影响软膏剂的质量及药物疗效的发挥，基质本身又有保护与润滑皮肤的作用。软膏基质可分为油脂性基质、水溶性基质和乳剂型基质。乳剂型基质可分为水包油型（O/W）和油包水型（W/O）。软膏剂、乳膏剂基质应根据剂型特点、药物性质、制剂疗效和产品稳定性进行选择。

软膏剂可采用研磨法、熔融法制备，乳膏剂采用乳化法制备，必要时可加入透皮吸收促进剂、保湿剂、防腐剂等附加剂。固体药物可用基质中的适当组分溶解，或先粉碎成细粉与少量基质或液体组分研成糊状，再与其他基质研匀。所制得的软膏剂、乳膏剂应均匀、细腻，具有适当的黏稠性，易涂于皮肤或黏膜上且无刺激性。软膏剂、乳膏剂在存放过程中应无酸败、异臭、变色、变硬、油水分离等变质现象发生。

软膏剂、乳膏剂中药物的释放及透皮吸收不仅与药物本身的性质相关，基质也会在一定程度上影响药物的释放或透皮特性。一般情况下，水溶性基质和乳剂型基质中药物的释放较快，烃类基质中的药物释放较慢。

药物从基质中释放有多种测定方法，如琼脂凝胶扩散法和 Franz 扩散法等。琼脂凝胶扩散法是用琼脂凝胶（有时也可用明胶）作为扩散介质，将软膏剂、乳膏剂涂在含有指示剂的凝胶表面，当药物分子进入琼脂凝胶中，就与琼脂凝胶中的指示剂起反应显色，通过测量药物与指示剂产生的色层高度可获得药物的释放速度。指示剂根据具体药物选择,如水杨酸的释放选择三氯化铁为指示剂。扩散距离与时间的关系可以用 Lockie 经验式 [式 (3 – 10 – 1)] 表示

$$H^2 = Kt \qquad\qquad (3 - 10 - 1)$$

式中,H 为扩散距离(单位为 mm),t 为扩散时间(单位为 h),K 为扩散系数(单位为 mm^2/h)。以不同时间色层高度的平方(H^2)对扩散时间(t)作图,可得到一条直线。此直线的斜率 K 即为扩散系数,K 反映软膏剂的释药速度。

琼脂凝胶法并不能模拟药物在皮肤中的吸收。体外经皮渗透实验则是经皮给药制剂开发中必不可少的研究手段,它是将离体皮肤固定在扩散池中,角质层面向供给池,然后将药物置于供给池中,经一定时间测定皮肤另一侧接收池内介质中的药物浓度。体外经皮渗透实验可以研究基质、处方组成和经皮吸收促进剂等对药物经皮渗透速率的影响,以及预测药物经皮吸收速度等,对研究经皮给药制剂具有重要价值。透皮渗透试验仪的构造及使用方法详见附录 IF。

三、预习思考

(1) 软膏剂、乳膏剂的质量要求有哪些?
(2) 软膏剂、乳膏剂常用基质的分类及其选择依据?

四、实验材料

1. 实验试剂与试药

水杨酸、蜂蜡、植物油、白凡士林、月桂醇硫酸钠、硬脂醇、甘油、液状石蜡、羧甲基纤维素钠、尼泊金乙酯、无水乙醇、琼脂、氯化铁、硫酸铁铵、盐酸、生理盐水、蒸馏水。

2. 实验仪器

天平、药匙、称量纸、滴管、烧杯、玻璃棒、蒸发皿、恒温水浴箱、量筒、研钵、试管、纱布、保鲜膜、直尺、搅拌子、一次性注射器、0.45 μm 微孔滤膜、紫外 – 分光光度计、透皮扩散试验仪。

五、实验内容

(一) 不同类型基质的制备

1. 油脂性基质 (单软膏)

(1) 处方:

蜂蜡	4.0 g
植物油	15.0 g

（2）实验步骤：

采用熔融法制备。取处方量蜂蜡于蒸发皿，70～80 ℃水浴加热熔化，缓慢加入植物油，搅拌均匀。放置室温下搅拌至冷凝，即得。

注意事项

加入植物油后应不断搅拌使混匀，然后从水浴取下放置室温搅拌至冷凝。如果冷凝过程中不搅拌则容易分层。

2. O/W 型基质

（1）处方：

硬脂醇	1.8 g
白凡士林	2.0 g
液状石蜡	1.3 mL
月桂醇硫酸钠	0.2 g
尼泊金乙酯	0.02 g
甘油	1.0 g
蒸馏水	15.0 g

（2）实验步骤：

采用乳化法制备。取油相（硬脂醇、白凡士林和液状石蜡）于蒸发皿中，置70～80 ℃水浴上加热；取水相（月桂醇硫酸钠、尼泊金乙酯、甘油和蒸馏水）于小烧杯中，置70～80 ℃水浴上加热。搅拌下将水相以细流状加入油相中，在70～80 ℃水浴中继续搅拌5 min，待乳化完全，放置室温下搅拌至冷凝，即得。

注意事项

水相、油相混合后沿一个方向搅拌，否则难以得到合格的乳剂型基质。

3. 水溶性基质

（1）处方：

羧甲基纤维素钠	1.2 g
甘油	3.0 g
尼泊金乙酯	0.02 g
蒸馏水	15 mL

（2）实验操作：

采用研磨法制备。取羧甲基纤维素钠于研钵中，加入处方量甘油，边研磨边缓缓加入约 15 mL 水，研匀得基质。将处方量尼泊金乙酯溶于约 1 mL 无水乙醇，加入已经制备的基质中，研匀即得。

（二）水杨酸软膏的制备

称取上述三种基质各 9.5 g，分别加入 0.5 g 水杨酸细粉，研磨均匀制得三种水杨酸软膏。

（三）水杨酸软膏中药物释放的测定（琼脂凝胶法）

称取琼脂 2 g，加水 100 mL，煮沸 10 min 使其溶解，经纱布粗滤后加入 1 mL 氯化铁试液，搅拌均匀后一次性注入试管中，注入高度以距管口约 1 cm 为宜（每种基质 1 支试管）。待琼脂冷却凝固后，将含药软膏小心转移至琼脂凝胶上端，使厚度约 1 cm，并与琼脂紧密接触。用保鲜膜将试管开口处封口密闭，分别于 1 h、2 h、4 h、6 h、8 h、24 h（可根据学生实验进度适当调整时间点）测定琼脂区呈色区高度 H。

（四）水杨酸软膏经皮渗透系数的测定

1. 水杨酸的含量测定

（1）硫酸铁铵显色剂配制：称取 8 g 硫酸铁铵溶于 100 mL 蒸馏水中，备用。取硫酸铁铵溶液 2 mL 和 1 mol/L 的盐酸溶液 1 mL，加蒸馏水定容至 100 mL，即得。

（2）标准曲线绘制：精密称取水杨酸对照品约 10 mg，用蒸馏水配制约 100 μg/mL 的水杨酸贮备液。取上述贮备液适量，经稀释配成浓度分别约为 5 μg/mL、10 μg/mL、20 μg/mL、40 μg/mL、80 μg/mL 的标准溶液。分别精密量取不同浓度的标准溶液 7.5 mL，加硫酸铁铵显色剂 1 mL，以蒸馏水 7.5 mL 加硫酸铁铵显色剂 1 mL 为空白，于紫外 – 可见光分光光度计 530 nm 处测定吸光度 A，将吸光度 A 对水杨酸浓度回归得标准曲线方程。

（3）经皮渗透实验。将鼠皮固定于扩散池中，供给池中加入不同基质的水杨酸软膏和空白基质各约 300 mg。接收池中加入生理盐水 7.5 mL，整个装置于（32±1）℃的水浴下保温，磁力搅拌器速度为 250 r/min。分别于 1 h、2 h、4 h、8 h、12 h、24 h 取出接收池样品 7.5 mL，并立即加入等量（32±1）℃ 生理盐水。样品经 0.45 μm 微孔滤膜过滤，适当稀释后，精密量取稀释液 7.5 mL，加硫酸铁铵显色剂 1 mL，于 530 nm 处测定吸光度。按标准曲线法计算接收介质中水杨酸的浓度。

2. 累积渗透量的计算

计算单位面积累积皮肤渗透量 Q，计算公式如式（3 – 10 – 2）：

$$Q = \left(C_n V + \sum_{i=1}^{n-1} C_i V_i \right) / A \qquad (3-10-2)$$

式中，A 为接收池面积；V 为接收介质体积；V_i 为每次取样体积，C_i 为第 i 次实测药物浓度，$i = 1, 2, \cdots, n$；Q 为完成第 n 次取样时水杨酸软膏、乳膏单位面积的累积渗透量。

3. 稳态渗透速率的计算

以单位面积累积渗透量 Q 对时间 t 作图得水杨酸的经皮渗透曲线，将渗透曲线直线部分的数据进行线性回归，求得直线斜率即为稳态渗透速率 J ［单位为 $\mu g/(cm^2 \cdot h)$］。

注意事项

（1）含指示剂的琼脂溶液应新鲜配制，为避免产生气泡，配制切勿剧烈搅拌，溶液中的少量气泡可在 60 ℃ 水浴中静置除去。

（2）含指示剂的琼脂溶液倾入试管时，温度不宜过高并应保持试管垂直，以免冷却后体积收缩，在试管内形成凹面或斜面，改变药物扩散面积。

（3）琼脂凝胶法测定药物释放时软膏、乳膏的装量应保持一致，且与琼脂凝胶的接触面以及制剂内部均不得留有空隙和气泡。

（4）硫酸铁铵显色剂应新鲜配制。

（5）接收池中的接收液注意要密切接触皮肤，并尽可能排尽与皮肤接触界面的气泡。

六、实验结果与讨论

（1）将制备得到的 3 种水杨酸软膏、乳膏涂抹在自己的手背皮肤上，评价是否均匀、细腻。比较 3 种软膏、乳膏的稠度与涂抹性。讨论 3 种软膏中各组分的作用。

（2）药物释放（琼脂凝胶法）。记录 1 h、2 h、4 h、8 h、12 h、24 h 呈色区高度 H。以 H^2 对 t 作图，斜率为药物扩散系数。分析不同基质对药物释放的影响。

将测得的结果填入表 3 - 38 中。

表 3 - 38　琼脂凝胶法测定水杨酸软膏的扩散系数

时间/h	处方 1		处方 2		处方 3	
	H/mm	H^2/mm^2	H/mm	H^2/mm^2	H/mm	H^2/mm^2
1						
2						
4						
8						
12						
24						
$H^2 - t$ 方程 扩散系数 K						

（3）药物经皮渗透系数的测定。记录在 1 h、2 h、4 h、8 h、12 h、24 h 时样品在 530 nm 处的吸光度，按标准曲线法计算接收介质中水杨酸的浓度。按式（3 - 10 - 2）计算单位面积累积渗透量 Q，以单位面积累积渗透量对时间 t 作图得水杨酸的经皮渗透曲线，将渗透曲线直线部分的数据进行线性回归，求得直线斜率即为稳态渗透速率

$J\left[\mu\mathrm{g}/(\mathrm{cm}^2\cdot\mathrm{h})\right]$。将测得的结果填入表 3-39 中。

表 3-39 水杨酸软膏的经皮渗透系数的测定

时间/h	处方 1		处方 2		处方 3	
	吸光度 A	浓度/ $(\mu\mathrm{g}\cdot\mathrm{mL}^{-1})$	吸光度 A	浓度/ $(\mu\mathrm{g}\cdot\mathrm{mL}^{-1})$	吸光度 A	浓度/ $(\mu\mathrm{g}\cdot\mathrm{mL}^{-1})$
1						
2						
4						
6						
8						
24						
累积渗透量 Q						
$Q-t$ 方程						
渗透速率 $J/\left[\mu\mathrm{g}\cdot(\mathrm{cm}^{-2}\cdot\mathrm{h})\right]$						

七、思考题

(1) 药物从不同基质的软膏剂中释放有何特点?

(2) 乳膏剂与乳剂在组成方面有何不同?

(3) 影响软膏剂、乳膏剂中药物释放的因素有哪些?

Experiment 10　Preparation of Ointments and Creams

Ⅰ. Purpose

(1) To master the components and preparation of different types of ointment bases.

(2) To be familiar with the methods to measure drug release from ointments and the effect of bases on drug release.

Ⅱ. Principles

Ointments are uniform semi-solid preparations made of drugs and oleaginous or water-soluble bases and are intended for external use. They can serve as therapeutic agents, protectants or emollients for the skin at the application site, and drugs can be absorbed into the systemic circulation to induce systemic therapeutic effects. According to different dispersion states of drugs in the bases, ointments are divided into solution type ointments and suspension type ointments. Solution type ointments are the ointments in which drug substances are dissolved or melted into single or compound bases; suspension type ointments are the ointments in which fine powders of drugs are evenly dispersed into the bases.

Creams are uniform semi-solid preparations made of emulsified bases in which drugs are dissolved or dispersed.

Bases are excipients for ointments and creams, which can endow ointments with certain characteristics and influence the quality and efficacy of ointments. Also, bases themselves can protect or moisturize the skin. Bases can be divided into oleaginous, water-soluble and emulsion bases. Emulsion bases can be further divided into oil-in-water (O/W) and water-in-oil (W/O) types. Bases utilized for ointments and creams are usually selected based on the types of dosage forms, the properties of drugs, the proposed efficacy and stability of preparations.

Ointments can be prepared by the methods of grinding or melting, and creams by emulsifying. If necessary, transdermal absorption enhancers, wetting agents and preservatives can be added to ointments and creams. Solid drugs can either be dissolved in appropriate components of bases, or be ground into fine powders and then mixed with a small amount of bases or its liquid components to form a paste before blended with the rest of bases. The prepared ointments and creams should be uniform, fine and smooth with proper viscosity, and easily applied to the skin and mucosa without any irritation. During storage, ointments and creams should show no appearance of deterioration such as rancidity, foreign odor, discoloration, hardening, and separation of oil and water.

Among quality inspections of ointments and creams, drug release is an important item. The drug release and transdermal absorption of ointments and creams are not only related to the properties of drugs but also influenced by their bases. In general, drugs release more quickly from water-soluble bases and emulsion bases than from oleaginous bases.

To assay drug release from bases, there are various methods such as agar gel diffusion method and Franz diffusion method. The agar gel diffusion method utilizes solid agar gel (sometimes gelatin) containing indicators as diffusion medium, on the surface of which ointments and creams are added. When drug molecules diffuse into the agar gel, they react with the indicators and display specific color. The drug release rate can be estimated by the height of the coloration zone. Indicators are selected according to the properties of drugs. For example, ferric trichloride is chosen to assay the release of salicylic acid. The relationship between diffusion distance and time is shown in the Lockie's empirical formula [formula (3 – 10 – 1)]:

$$H^2 = Kt \qquad\qquad (3 - 10 - 1)$$

In this formula, H is the diffusion distance (mm); t is the diffusion time (h); K is the diffusion coefficient (mm^2/h). Plotting the square of the height of coloration zones (H^2) against diffusion time (t) obtains a resulting straight line, the slope rate of which is the diffusion coefficient K, reflecting the drug release rate of ointments.

However, agar gel diffusion method can not mimic the drug absorption through the skin well. The *in vitro* percutaneous penetration test is an indispensable method for development of the transdermal drug delivery system. In this method, isolated skin is fixed in the diffusion cell and its stratum corneum faces the donor cell, then the drug is added to the donor cell and semisolid preparations spread evenly on the skin. After a certain period of time, drug concentrations in the receptor cell on the other side of the skin can be determined. In this way, the effects of bases and percutaneous absorption enhancers on the percutaneous penetration can be investigated, which is of great value for research on transdermal preparations. See Appendix ⅠF for detailed instructions of percutaneous permeation apparatus.

Ⅲ. Preview

(1) What are the quality requirements of ointments and creams?

(2) Please describe the classification of bases utilized for ointments and creams and the selection principles.

Ⅳ. Experiment materials and equipments

1. Reagents and experimental materials

Salicylic acid, beeswax, vegetable oil, white vaseline, sodium lauryl sulfate, stearic alcohol, glycerol, liquid paraffin, sodium carboxymethyl cellulose, ethyl paraben, agar, ferric chloride, ammonium ferric sulfate, hydrochloric acid, saline, distilled water.

2. Experimental equipments

Balance, ultraviolet spectrophotometer, transdermal diffusion instrument, evaporating dish, constant temperature water bath, grinding bowl, screen, test tube, ruler, disposable syringe, 0.45 μm microporous filter.

Ⅴ. Experiment contents

1. Preparation of different types of bases

1) Oleaginous bases (single ointments):

(1) Formulation:

Beeswax	4.0 g
Vegetable oil	15.0 g

(2) Procedures:

Oleaginous bases are prepared by melting method. Put the required mass of beeswax in an evaporating dish, and heat it in water bath at $70 \sim 80$ ℃ until melted. Then, slowly add vegetable oil to the melted beeswax under stirring. Remove the mixture from the water bath and keep stirring until concretion to obtain the oleaginous bases.

[Precautions]

After adding vegetable oil, keep stirring until the mixture condenses, otherwise it will easily become layered and unevenly mixed.

2) Oil-in-water bases:

(1) Formulation:

Stearic alcohol	1.8 g
White vaseline	2.0 g
Liquid paraffin	1.3 mL
Sodium lauryl sulfate	0.2 g
Ethyl paraben	0.02 g
Glycerol	1.0 g
Distilled water	15.0 g

(2) Procedures:

Oil-in-water bases are prepared by emulsification method. Put the oil phase (composed of stearic alcohol, white vaseline and liquid paraffin) in an evaporating dish, and heat it to 70 ~ 80 ℃ in water bath. Put the water phase (composed of sodium lauryl sulfate, ethyl paraben, glycerol and distilled water) in a beaker, and heat it to 70 ~ 80 ℃ in water bath. Add the water phase into the oil phase in a trickle, and keep stirring until emulsification. Continue to stir for 5 minutes in water bath at 70 ~ 80 ℃, and then place it at room temperature keeping stirring until condensation to obtain oil-in-water bases.

[Precautions]

After mixing water phase with oil phase, keep stirring in one direction, otherwise it will be hard to obtain a qualified emulsion base.

3) Water-soluble bases:

(1) Formulation:

Sodium carboxymethyl cellulose	1.2 g
Glycerol	3.0 g
Ethyl paraben	0.02 g
Distilled water	15 mL

(2) Procedures:

Water-soluble bases are prepared by grinding method. Take sodium carboxymethyl cellulose in the mortar, add the prescribed amount of glycerin, then slowly add about 15 mL of water under grinding until uniform. Dissolve the prescribed amount of ethyl paraben in about 1 mL of ethanol and add to the mixture above to obtain the water-soluble bases.

2. Preparation of salicylic acid ointments

Weigh the above three bases 9.5 g respectively, add 0.5 g of salicylic acid powders and mix evenly to obtain three types of salicylic acid ointments.

3. Drug release in salicylic acid ointments (agar gel method)

Put 2 g of agar in 100 mL of water and boil for 10 minutes until agar dissolves. After filtering the solution through a piece of gauze, mix the solution with 1 mL of ferric chloride solution, then inject the gar solution into test tube until $1 \sim 2$ cm above the tube orifice (1 tube for each type of base). After the agar is cooled down and solidified, carefully transfer salicylic acid ointments with 1-cm-thick to the upper end of the agar gel and make the agar and ointments in close contact. Seal the test tube with a cling film. Test the height (H) of coloration zone in the agar region at 1 h, 2 h, 4 h, 6 h, 8 h and 24 h (The time point can be moderately adjusted according to students' experiment progress) after loading.

4. Determination of permeation coefficient of salicylic acid ointments

1) Determination of salicylic acid content:

(1) Preparation of ammonium ferric sulfate reagents:

Weigh 8 g of ammonium ferric sulfate and dissolve it in 100 mL of distilled water. Mix 2 mL of the ammonium ferric sulfate solution with 1 mL of the hydrochloric acid solution (1 mol/L), and add distilled water up to 100 mL.

(2) Charting of the standard curve:

Precisely weigh about 10 mg of salicylic acid reference substance and dissolve in distilled water to form a salicylic acid solution of 100 μg/mL. Dilute the salicylic acid solution to prepare standard solution of approximately 5 μg/mL, 10 μg/mL, 20 μg/mL, 40 μg/mL and 80 μg/mL, respectively.

Precisely measure 7.5 mL of each standard solution with different concentrations, and add 1 mL of the ammonium ferric sulfate reagent to each solution. Measure 7.5 mL of distilled water, and add 1 mL of the ammonium ferric sulfate reagent to prepare a blank solution.

Determine the absorbance (A) of each solution at 530 nm through an ultraviolet-visible spectrophotometer, and regress the absorbance (A) to the concentration of salicylic acid to obtain the calibration curve equation.

(3) Percutaneous penetration test:

Fix rat skin in a diffusion cell. Add about 300 mg of blank bases and salicylic acid ointments with different bases to the donor cell. Add 7.5 mL of physiological saline to the receptor cell, and keep the whole device in a water bath at (32 ± 1) ℃ while fixing the speed of the magnetic stirrer at 250 r/min. At 1 h, 2 h, 4 h, 8 h, 12 h and 24 h after addition, withdraw 7.5 mL of receiving medium from the receptor cell, and immediately replenish an equal amount (7.5 mL) of fresh physiological saline at (32 ± 1) ℃. Filter the receiving medium through

0. 45 μm microporous membrane. After appropriate dilution, precisely measure 7. 5 mL of the diluted sample and add 1 mL of the ammonium ferric sulfate reagent, measure the absorbance of the solution at 530 nm. Calculate the concentration of salicylic acid in the receiving medium by the calibration curve method.

2) Calculation of the cumulative transdermal dosage:

Calculate the cumulative transdermal amount per unit area (Q) according to the formula (3 – 10 – 2):

$$Q = (C_n V + \sum_{i=1}^{n-1} C_i V_i)/A \qquad (3 - 10 - 2)$$

In this formula, A is the area of the receptor cell; V is the volume of the receiving medium; V_i is the volume of each sample; C_i is the measured drug concentration at the i th time ($i = 1$, 2, ..., n); Q is the cumulative transdermal amount per unit area of salicylic acid ointments or creams when achieving the n th sampling.

3) Calculation of the steady-state penetration rate:

Obtain the transdermal permeation curve of salicylic acid by plotting the cumulative permeation per unit area (Q) against time (t), and regress the data drawn from the linear part of the transdermal permeation curve. The slope rate of the resulting line is the steady-state penetration rate J [μg/(cm^2 · h)].

[Precautions]

(1) The agar solution containing indicators should be freshly prepared. To avoid bubbles, vigorous stirring should be avoided during the preparation process. A small number of bubbles in the solution can be removed by leaving it in a water bath at 60 ℃.

(2) When the agar solution containing indicators is poured into the test tube, the temperature should not be too high in order to avoid volume contraction after cooling down. The test tube should be kept perpendicular to avoid the formation of concave or inclined surface in the test tube which could alter the drug diffusion area.

(3) When the agar gel method is used to measure the drug release from ointments and creams, the amount of ointments and creams should be kept consistent and there should be no gaps or bubbles inside the ointments or creams or in the interface between the agar gel and ointments or creams.

(4) The ammonium ferric sulfate reagent should be freshly prepared.

(5) The receiving fluid in the receptor cell should be in close contact with the skin, and the air bubbles in contact with the skin interface should be exhausted as far as possible.

VI. Experiment results and discussion

(1) Apply three prepared salicylic acid ointments and creams on the back skin of your hand to evaluate whether they are uniform, fine and smooth. Compare the consistency and

spread ability of three ointments and creams, and discuss the roles of each component in the three ointments.

(2) Drug release (agar gel method). Record the height of the coloration zones (H) at 1 h, 2 h, 4 h, 8 h, 12 h and 24 h after the addition of ointments. The slope rate of the H^2 to t is drug diffusion coefficient. Analyze the effects of different bases on drug release. Fill the result in Table 3 – 38.

Table 3 – 38   Diffusion coefficient of salicylic acid ointments (agar gel method)

t/h	F1		F2		F3	
	H/mm	H^2/mm^2	H/mm	H^2/mm^2	H/mm	H^2/mm^2
1						
2						
4						
6						
8						
24						
$H^2 - t$ equation K						

(3) Determination of transdermal permeation coefficient. Record the absorbance of receiving medium at 530 nm at 1 h, 2 h, 4 h, 8 h, 12 h, 24 h after the addition of ointments. Calculate the concentration of salicylic acid in the receiving medium by the calibration curve method. Calculate the cumulative penetration volume per unit area (Q) based on the formula (3 – 10 – 2). Plot Q to time (t) to obtain the permeability curve of salicylic acid, and regress the data drawn from the linear part of the curve. The slope rate of the resulting line is the steady-state penetration rate J [μg/(cm^2 · h)]. Fill the result in Table 3 – 39.

Table 3 – 39   Transdermal permeation coefficient of salicylic acid ointments

t/h	F1		F2		F3	
	Abs	c/(μg · mL^{-1})	Abs	c/(μg · mL^{-1})	Abs	c/(μg · mL^{-1})
1						
2						
4						
8						
12						
24						
Q						
$Q - t$ equation						
J/ [μg/(cm^{-2} · h)]						

VII. Questions

（1）What are the differences in drug release from ointments and creams with different bases?

（2）What are the differences between creams and emulsions in components?

（3）Discuss the actors influencing drug release from ointments and creams based on experiment results.

实验十一 栓剂的制备

一、实验目的

（1）掌握热熔法制备栓剂的方法。

（2）掌握置换价测定方法及应用。

（3）熟悉栓剂的质量检查方法。

二、实验原理

栓剂（suppositories）系指原料药物与适宜基质制成的可供腔道给药的半固体制剂。其形状和大小根据腔道不同而异。目前临床上常用的有直肠栓和阴道栓等。

栓剂应外形完整光滑、无刺激性且具有一定硬度，其熔点应接近体温，置入腔道后应能熔融、软化或溶解，释放出药物产生局部或全身作用。

栓剂中药物的释放行为受基质影响较大。栓剂的基质可分为油脂性基质和水溶性基质（亲水性基质）两类。前者如可可豆脂、半合成脂肪酸酯等，后者如甘油明胶、聚乙二醇类、聚氧乙烯脂肪酸酯类等。此外，在基质中加入适量表面活性剂可促进药物释放和吸收。

栓剂的制备方法有冷压法和热熔法，可根据基质的性质选择不同的制备方法。油脂性基质制备的栓剂可以用冷压法和热熔法制备，水溶性基质则多采用热熔法。

热熔法制备栓剂的工艺流程如图 3 – 12 所示。

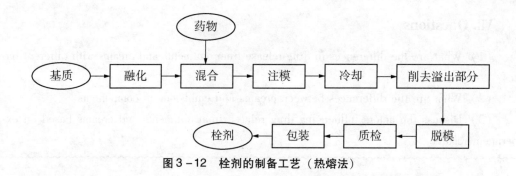

图3-12 栓剂的制备工艺（热熔法）

为保证栓剂剂量的准确，应预先测定药物的置换价（displacement value，DV）以确定栓剂所需基质的用量。置换价指药物质量与同体积栓剂基质的质量比。

根据式（3-11-1）计算DV，

$$DV = \frac{W}{[G - (M - W)]} \qquad (3-11-1)$$

其中，G为纯基质栓的平均质量，M为测定置换价时所用的含药栓的平均质量，W为含药栓的平均含药量；药物含量为C%的含药栓，每枚含药栓的平均含药量为 $W = M \times C\%$。根据置换价，代入式（3-11-2），可计算出含药栓所需基质的质量E。

$$E = G - \frac{W^*}{DV} \qquad (3-11-2)$$

其中，W^* 表示栓剂处方中药物的标示量。

为了让栓剂容易脱模，注模前可在模具表面涂抹适量的润滑剂。其中油脂性基质一般选择水溶性润滑剂，常用的是软皂-甘油-95%乙醇体积比为1:1:5混合液；水溶性基质一般选用液状石蜡或硅油等油溶性润滑剂。

栓剂为供腔道给药的制剂，应在洁净环境中制备。所需用具和容器应充分清洁或消毒，原料和基质也应符合相应的卫生学要求。

栓剂的质量检查包括外观性状、重量差异、融变时限、释放度、含量测定及微生物限度等。

三、预习思考

（1）理想的栓剂基质应符合哪些要求？
（2）栓剂基质的选用依据有哪些？不同基质栓剂的处方设计应考虑哪些因素？
（3）思考测定栓剂融变时限的意义。

四、实验材料与仪器

1. 实验试剂与试药

吲哚美辛、半合成脂肪酸酯、甲硝唑、醋酸氯己定、聚山梨酯80、冰片、乙醇、甘油、明胶、聚氧乙烯（40）单硬脂酸酯（S-40）、枸橼酸、碳酸氢钠、无水氯化钙、软皂乙醇液、液体石蜡、蒸馏水。

2. 实验仪器

天平、恒温水浴锅、电加热套、烘箱、栓剂模具、融变时限检查仪、药匙、称量纸、蒸发皿、玻璃棒、刮铲、研钵、筛网、烧杯、量筒、具塞刻度试管等。

五、实验内容

（一）吲哚美辛栓

1. 纯基质栓的制备

取 10 g 半合成脂肪酸酯于蒸发皿中，水浴加热至 2/3 基质熔化，停止加热。搅拌使其全熔，稍冷，注入涂有软皂乙醇液（润滑剂）的栓剂模具内。冷却，削去模口溢出部分。脱模，称量取平均值，得 G。

2. 含药栓的制备

（1）处方：

吲哚美辛（100 目）	1 g
半合成脂肪酸酯	10 g

（2）实验步骤：取半合成脂肪酸酯于蒸发皿中，水浴加热至 2/3 基质熔化，停止加热，搅拌使其全熔。分次缓慢加入吲哚美辛细粉（预先过 100 目筛），迅速搅拌均匀。稍冷，注入涂有软皂乙醇液的模具内。冷却，削去模口溢出部分。脱模、称重取平均值，得 M，计算栓剂中药物的含量 W。

根据式（11-1）计算吲哚美辛与半合成脂肪酸酯的置换价 DV。根据吲哚美辛栓的标示量 $W^* = 100$ mg 计算 10 粒含药栓所需基质的量 $10E$。

3. 吲哚美辛栓剂的制备

（1）处方：

吲哚美辛（100 目）	1 g
半合成脂肪酸酯	10E
制成	10 粒

（2）实验步骤：

参照"2. 含药栓的制备"步骤，制备吲哚美辛栓。

对吲哚美辛栓进行外观性状、分散状态、重量差异以及融变时限检查。

注意事项

（1）基质熔化加入药物至注模，应保持搅拌防止药物沉降，避免药物含量不均匀。

（2）注模时，基质应保持温度适宜。温度太高则基质与药物不易混合均匀，栓剂易发生中空或顶端凹陷；温度太低则基质黏稠，难以一次性注模成功。

（3）注模后，模具应置于适宜的温度下，等待完全冷却后才削去溢出部分。冷却温度过低易导致栓剂破碎；冷却时间不足则易发生黏膜，无法得到完整栓剂。

（4）为保证置换价测定的准确性，制备纯基质栓和含药栓时应采用同一模具。

（二）醋酸氯己定栓（洗必泰）

1. 处方

醋酸氯己定	0.25 g
聚山梨酯 80	1.0 g
冰片	0.05 g
乙醇	2.5 g
甘油	32 g
明胶	9 g
蒸馏水加至	50 g

2. 实验步骤

（1）甘油明胶溶液的制备。称取处方量的明胶，置蒸发皿中。加入相当于明胶质量 1.5～2.0 倍的蒸馏水浸泡 0.5～1.0 h。充分溶胀后，加入处方量甘油，水浴加热。待明胶溶解，继续加热并轻轻搅拌，使水分蒸发至溶液约 46 g 为止。

（2）栓剂的制备。将醋酸氯己定与聚山梨酯 80 混匀。冰片溶于乙醇中，并加至醋酸氯己定混合物中，持续搅拌至均匀。将其加至上述甘油明胶溶液中，保持搅拌。趁热灌入已涂有液体石蜡（润滑剂）的栓模内，冷却，削去模口上的溢出部分。脱模，质检，包装，即得。

对醋酸氯己定栓进行外观性状、分散状态、重量差异以及融变时限检查。

注意事项

比例不同的甘油、明胶和水可制得硬度不同的栓剂基质。实验中应严格控制水量，以确保栓剂硬度适中。

（三）甲硝唑泡腾栓

1. 处方

甲硝唑	2 g
S-40	17.5 g
枸橼酸	2 g
碳酸氢钠	2.5 g
制成	10 粒

2. 实验步骤

将干燥的枸橼酸和碳酸氢钠分别研细，过 60 目筛放置干燥器中备用。S-40 用电热套加热熔融，加约 3 g 无水氯化钙并搅拌脱水，静置 2～3 min。将基质转移至烧杯（注意避免倾出氯化钙），置电热套中保温（约 50 ℃）维持熔融状态。在搅拌下加入甲硝唑细粉、枸橼酸和碳酸氢钠，混合均匀。趁热倾入涂有液体石蜡的模具中，冷却，脱模即得。

对所制得栓剂进行外观性状、分散状态、重量差异以及发泡量实验检查。

注意事项

（1）该处方中的枸橼酸和碳酸氢钠为泡腾剂，使用时应处于干燥状态。临用前将枸橼酸置于 105 ℃干燥 2 h，碳酸氢钠置于 55 ℃干燥 2 h。

（2）泡腾栓的基质熔融时要用电热套加热，避免水蒸气的带入。

（3）制备泡腾栓时药物及泡腾剂的加入要迅速，防止泡腾剂吸潮，影响泡腾结果。

六、实验结果与讨论

1. 外观性状与分散状态

栓剂外形应完整光滑，硬度适宜，无变形，无斑点和气泡。将栓剂纵向剖开，观察药物分散是否均匀。

2. 重量差异

取制得的栓剂 10 粒，精密称定总质量，求得平均粒重后，再分别精密称定每粒的质量。比较每粒质量与平均粒重（有标示粒重的中药栓剂，每粒质量应与标示粒重比较）。按表 3-40 中的规定，超出重量差异限度的不得多于 1 粒，并不得超出限度 1 倍。将检查结果填入表 3-41 至表 3-43 中。

表3-40 栓剂重量差异限度

平均粒重或标示粒重	重量差异限度
1.0 g 及 1.0 g 以下	±10%
1.0 g 以上至 3.0 g	±7.5%
3.0 g 以上	±5%

表3-41 吲哚美辛栓重量差异检查结果

编号	1	2	3	4	5	6	7	8	9	10	平均质量/g
吲哚美辛栓/g											
重量差异范围/g											
结论											

表3-42 醋酸氯己定栓重量差异检查结果

编号	1	2	3	4	5	6	7	8	9	10	平均质量/g
醋酸氯己定栓/g											
重量差异范围/g											
结论											

表3-43 甲硝唑泡腾栓重量差异检查结果

编号	1	2	3	4	5	6	7	8	9	10	平均质量/g
甲硝唑泡腾栓/g											
重量差异范围/g											
结论											

3. 融变时限检查

除另有规定外,参照融变时限检查法(2020 版《中国药典》通则 0922)进行检查。取供试品 3 粒,室温放置 1 h 后,分别放在融变时限检查仪 3 个金属架的下层圆板上,装入各自的套筒内,并用挂钩固定,融变时限检查仪的使用见附录 IJ。除另有规定外,将上述装置分别垂直浸入盛有不少于 4 L 的 (37.0 ±0.5) ℃ 水的容器中,其上端位置应在水面下 90 mm 处。容器中装有转动器,每隔 10 min 在溶液中翻转套筒 1 次。除另有规定外,3 粒油脂性基质的栓剂均应在 30 min 内全部熔化、软化或触压无硬心;3 粒水溶性基质的栓剂均应在 60 min 内全部溶解。如有 1 粒不符合规定,应另取 3 粒复试,均应符合规定。将检查结果填入表3-44、表3-45 中。

表 3 – 44　吲哚美辛栓的融变时限检查结果

编号	1	2	3
融变时限/min			
结论			

表 3 – 45　醋酸氯己定栓的融变时限检查结果

编号	1	2	3
融变时限/min			
结论			

4. 甲硝唑泡腾栓发泡量的测定

观察并记录起泡时间、最大发泡量与起泡持续时间。取 25 mL 具塞刻度试管（内径约 1.5 cm）10 支，各精密加水 2 mL。置（37 ± 1）℃ 水浴中 5 min 后，各管中分别投入栓剂 1 枚，20 min 内观察最大发泡量的体积。平均发泡体积应不少于 10.0 mL，且少于 6.0 mL 的不应超过 2 枚。将检查结果填入表 3 – 46 中。

表 3 – 46　甲硝唑泡腾栓剂发泡量检查结果

编号	1	2	3	4	5	6	7	8	9	10	Mean ± SD
起泡时间/s											
最大发泡量/mL											
起泡持续时间/min											

七、思考题

（1）测定置换价对栓剂的制备有什么意义？

（2）吲哚美辛栓应优选哪类基质？为什么？

（3）吲哚美辛栓是起局部作用还是起全身作用？设计起全身作用的栓剂应考虑哪些因素？

Experiment 11　Preparation of Suppositories

Ⅰ. Purpose

(1) To master the preparation of suppositories by fusion method.

(2) To master measurement method and application of the displacement value.

(3) To be familiar with quality inspection methods of suppositories.

Ⅱ. Principles

Suppositories are semi-solid preparations comprised of active ingredients and suitable bases for cavity administration. Their shapes and sizes vary with the cavity application sites. At present, rectal suppositories and vaginal suppositories are commonly used in clinical treatments.

Suppositories should be complete in forms, smooth in appearances with moderate hardness and no irritation, and possess a melting point close to body temperature. After been placed into cavity, suppositories can be fused, softened or dissolved, and release drug then produce local or systemic effects.

Release properties of suppositories are greatly influenced by their bases. Bases of suppositories can be grouped into two categories: lipophilic and hydrophilic bases. The former contains cocoa butter, semi-synthetic fatty acid esters, etc. The latter consists of glycerin gelatin, polyethylene glycols, polyoxyethylene fatty acid esters and so on. Surfactants can also be added to promote drug release and absorption.

Preparation of suppositories includes cold compression method and fusion method. Various methods can be selected according to different bases. Suppositories, composed of lipophilic bases, can be prepared by cold compression method and fusion method, while suppositories composed of hydrophilic bases are mostly prepared by fusion method.

The steps for preparing suppositories by fusion method are as follows:

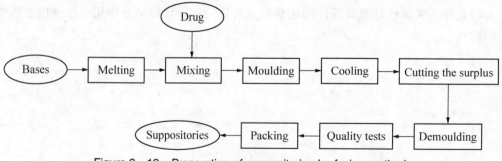

Figure 3 – 12　Preparation of suppositories by fusion method

In order to ensure accuracy of suppositories dosage, displacement value (DV) of drugs should be done first to determine the amount of base in suppositories. DV refers to weight ratio of drug to bases with the same volume in suppositories.

The calculation formula of DV is formula $(3-11-1)$:

$$DV = \frac{W}{[\,G - (M - W)\,]} \qquad (3-11-1)$$

G is the average weight of blank suppositories; M is the average weight of drug-loaded suppositories; W is the average drug content of suppositories, $W = M \times C\%$, where $C\%$ is drug content proportion in drug-loaded suppositories. E, the weight of the bases needed to prepare suppository, according to formula $(3-11-2)$, can be calculated conveniently by using DV:

$$E = G - \frac{W^*}{DV} \qquad (3-11-2)$$

W^* refers to the labeled amount of drug in suppositories.

In order to make suppositories easier to demold, a proper amount of lubricants is usually applied on mold surface before pouring. Water-soluble lubricants are generally employed for lipophilic bases, commonly using mixed solution of soft soap-glycerin-95% ethanol as $1:1:5$ $(V/V/V)$. Oil-soluble lubricants, such as liquid paraffin or silicone oil, are used for hydrophilic bases.

Suppositories, utilized for cavity administration, should be prepared in a cleanroom. Appliances and containers should be cleaned or disinfected enough. Ingredients and bases should meet the corresponding hygienic requirements.

Quality inspections of suppositories include appearance, weight variation, disintegration, release, content and microbial limit, etc.

III. Preview

(1) What requirements should the ideal bases of suppositories meet?

(2) What are the principles for selecting the suppositories bases? What factors should be considered during the formulation design of suppositories with various bases?

(3) What is the significance of performing disintegration test?

IV. Experiment materials and equipments

1. Reagents and experimental materials

Indomethacin, semi-synthetic fatty acid glyceride, metronidazole, chlorhexidine acetate, polysorbide 80, borneol, ethanol, glycerol, gelatin, polyethylene oxide (40) monostearate (S-40), citric acid, sodium bicarbonate, anhydrous $CaCl_2$, soft soap ethanol solution, liquid paraffin, distilled water.

2. Experimental equipments

Balance, thermostat water bath, heating mantle, oven, suppositories mold, disintegration test apparatus, spoon, weighing paper, evaporating dish, glass rod, scraper, grinding bowl, screen, beaker, graduated cylinder, graduated tube with plug, etc.

V. Experiment contents

1. Preparation of indomethacin suppositories

1) Preparation of blank suppositories.

Take 10 g of semi-synthetic fatty acid esters, place in the evaporating dish. Heat them in water bath until 2/3 of the bases are melted. Stop heating by removing the dish away from water bath, and keep stirring to make the bases fully melted. After the bases become slightly cool, pour them into suppositories mold, where soft soap ethanol liquid (lubricant) is pre-coated carefully on its surface. After the bases are cooled down, cut off the spilled part. Demold and weigh these blank suppositories to obtain average mass of suppositories G.

2) Preparation of drug-loaded suppositories.

(1) Formulation:

Indomethacin (100 mesh)	1 g
Semi-synthetic fatty acid esters	10 g

(2) Procedures:

Put the semi-synthetic fatty acid esters in the evaporating dish. Heat them in water bath until 2/3 of the bases are melted. Stop heating and keep stirring to make the bases fully melted. Indomethacin (filtered by 100 mesh sieve) is added slowly and stirred evenly. After the bases become slightly cool, pour it into suppositories mold, on whose surface soft soap ethanol liquid (lubricant) is pre-coated. When the bases are cooled down, cut off their spilled part. Demold and weigh the suppositories to get their average weight M. The content, W, in suppositories then is calculated.

DV of indomethacin to semi-synthetic fatty acid esters is calculated according to formula 11 − 1. Then, calculate the amount of bases needed for 10 suppositories ($10E$) according to the labeled amount of indomethacin suppositories $W^* = 100$ mg.

3) Preparation of indomethacin suppositories

(1) Formulation:

Indomethacin (100 mesh)	1 g
Semi-synthetic fatty acid esters	$10E$
Obtain	10 suppositories

2) Procedures:

Preparation of indomethacin suppositories as mentioned in 1. 2).

Appearance, dispersion, weight variation and disintegrating time of indomethacin suppositories should be examined.

[**Precautions**]

(1) After bases are melted and drug is added, keep stirring to avoid drug sedimentation and non-uniform distribution before suppositories are molded.

(2) Temperature is extremely important for successful molding and ideal shaping of suppositories. If temperature is excessive high, bases and drug can hardly mix well, and the suppositories are prone to be hollow or top collapse. If temperature is excessive low, bases will be too thick to finish molding for one time.

(3) After molding, mold should be completely cooled, and then cut off the spilled part. Excessive low temperature can easily lead to breakage of suppositories, while cooling time is insufficient, suppositories will easily stick to mold, resulting in fragmentary suppositories.

(4) To ensure accuracy of *DV* determination, the same mold should be utilized to prepare pure matrix and drug-loaded suppositories.

2. Preparation of chlorhexidine acetate suppositories

1) Formulation:

Chlorhexidine acetate	0.25 g
Polysorbide 80	1.0 g
Borneol	0.05 g
Ethanol	2.5 g
Glycerol	32 g
Gelatin	9 g
Distilled water added to	50 g

2) Procedures:

(1) Preparation of glycerin gelatin solution:

Required amount of gelatin is weighed and placed in an evaporating dish. Then gelatin is soaked in distilled water with the amount equal to 1.5 ~ 2.0 times of the gelatin for 0.5 ~ 1.0 h. After the gelatin is completely swelled, pre-heated glycerol should be added under gentle stirring and keep heating. Evaporate excessive water and get a mixture about 46 g.

(2) Preparation of suppositories:

Dissolve borneol in ethanol, and then add it to the mixture composed of chlorhexidine acetate and polysorbate 80 under gentle stirring. Then the mixture is poured into the glycerol gelatin solution under stirring. Before the bases cool down, pour them into suppositories mold, that liquid paraffin (lubricant) is pre-coated on the surface. When the bases are cooled down, cut off the spilled part. Demold and perform the quality inspections and package it.

（3）Appearance, dispersion, weight variation and disintegrating time of chlorhexidine acetate suppositories should be examined.

[**Precautions**]

Suppository bases with different hardness can be obtained through different proportions of glycerol, gelatin and water. The amount of water should be strictly controlled in order to ensure that hardness of suppositories is moderate.

3. Preparation of metronidazole effervescent suppositories

（1）Formulation：

Metronidazole	2 g
S- 40	17. 5 g
Citric acid	2 g
Sodium bicarbonate	2. 5 g
Obtain	10 suppositories

（2）Procedure：

Dried citric acid and sodium bicarbonate are ground separately, sieve through 60-mesh and place in a dryer for use. Heat S- 40 in an electric heater to become wholly melted, then add about 3 g of anhydrous $CaCl_2$ and slightly stir. Put it still for $2 \sim 3$ min to fully dehydrate. Transfer the melted base to a beaker and heat by an electronic heater (about 50 ℃) to remain the melting state. Metronidazole powder, citric acid and sodium bicarbonate are rapidly added under stirring. Before the bases cool down, pour them into suppositories mold, on whose surface liquid paraffin (lubricant) is pre-coated. When the bases are cooled down, cut off the spilled part. Demold and perform the quality inspections and package it.

Appearance, dispersion, weight variation and disintegrating time of metronidazole effervescent suppositories should be examined.

[**Precautions**]

（1）Citric acid and sodium bicarbonate here are effervescent agents. Before using, they must be in a dry state. Citric acid should be dried at 105 ℃ for 2 h and sodium bicarbonate should be dehydrated at 55 ℃ for 2 h.

（2）Electric heater rather than water bath should be utilized to melt bases in order to avoid absorption of moisture.

（3）When preparing effervescent suppositories, drug and effervescent agents should be quickly added, preventing effervescent agents from absorbing moisture.

VI. Experiment results and discussion

1. Appearance and dispersion

The shape of suppositories should be complete and smooth with suitable hardness and no deformation. There should be no spots and bubbles. Cut the suppositories lengthways to observe whether the drug is uniformly dispersed.

2. Weight variation

Ten suppositories are precisely weighed, and calculate the average weight. The weight of each suppository should be precisely weighed. Compare the weight of each suppository with the average weight (the weight of each suppository should be compared with the labeled weight if exhibited) according to requirements in Table 3 – 40. No more than one suppository should deviate from the average weight over the weight variation limit. Fill the result in Table 3 – 41 to Table 3 – 43.

Table 3 – 40　Weight variation limit

Average or labeled weight	Weight variation limit
1. 0 g or less	±10%
More than 1. 0 g to 3. 0 g	±7. 5%
More than 3. 0 g	±5%

Table 3 – 41　Weight variation of indomethacin suppositories

Number	1	2	3	4	5	6	7	8	9	10	Average weight/g
Indomethacin suppositories/g											
Qualified range of weight/g											
Conclusion											

Table 3 – 42　Weight variation of chlorhexidine acetate suppositories

Number	1	2	3	4	5	6	7	8	9	10	Average weight/g
Chlorhexidine acetate suppositories/g											
Qualified range of weight/g											
Conclusion											

Table 3 – 43　Weight variation of metronidazole effervescent suppositories

Number	1	2	3	4	5	6	7	8	9	10	Average weight/g
Metronidazole effervescent suppositories/g											
Qualified range of weight/g											
Conclusion											

3. Disintegration test

Unless otherwise stipulated, it should comply with the Disintegration Test (0922, ChP 2020). Three suppositories are stored at room temperature for 1 h. Then place them on the lower discs in their respective sleeves of the apparatus and fix them with hooks. Instructions for disintegration test machine are shown in Appendix ⅠJ. Unless otherwise specified, the above apparatus should be immersed vertically in containers containing water at (37.0 ± 0.5) ℃ of not less than 4 L, and located vertically 90 mm below water surface. A rotator is installed in the container, and the sleeve is inverted once every 10 min in the solution. Unless otherwise stipulated, all the three suppositories contained lipophilic bases should be melted, softened or contain no hard core within 30 min. All the three suppositories with hydrophilic bases should be dissolved within 60 min. If one does not meet the requirement, another three suppositories should be taken for re-examination. Fill the result in Table 3 – 44 and Table 3 – 45.

Table 3 – 44　Disintegration test of indomethacin suppositories

Number	1	2	3
Disintegrating time/min			
Conclusion			

Table 3 – 45　Disintegration test of chlorhexidine acetate suppositories

Number	1	2	3
Disintegrating time/min			
Conclusion			

4. Foaming quantity of metronidazole effervescent suppositories

The foaming time, maximum foaming volume and duration should be examined. Ten graduated tubes with plugs of 25 mL (inner diameter is about 1.5 cm) are selected. Add 2 mL of water respectively, and each tube is placed in water bath at (37.0 ± 1.0) ℃ for 5 min. Suppositories are put into the tubes respectively for 20 min. The maximum foaming volume should be no less than 10.0 mL on the average, and no more than 2 suppositories are less than 6.0 mL. Fill the result in Table 3 – 46.

Table 3-46 Foaming volume of metronidazole effervescent suppositories

Number	1	2	3	4	5	6	7	8	9	10	Mean ± SD
Foaming time/s											
Foaming volume/mL											
Duration/min											

VII. Questions

(1) Why is DV so significant for suppository preparations?

(2) What kind of bases should be employed in indomethacin suppositories? Give the reasons.

(3) Do indomethacin suppositories have local or systemic effects? What factors should be considered during suppositories' design for the systemic utilize?

实验十二 涂膜剂的制备

一、实验目的

(1) 掌握小量制备涂膜剂的方法。
(2) 熟悉常用成膜材料的性质与特点。
(3) 了解涂膜剂的质量评价方法。

二、实验原理

涂膜剂（pigments）是指药物溶解或分散在含成膜材料的溶剂中，涂擦患处后形成薄膜的外用液体制剂。涂膜剂溶剂挥发后形成的薄膜可保护患处，随后药物逐渐释放起治疗作用，一般用于无渗出液的皮肤表面。

涂膜剂通常由药物、成膜材料、挥发性溶剂和增塑剂等成分组成。常用的成膜材料有聚乙烯醇、聚乙烯吡咯烷酮、乙基纤维素和聚乙烯醇缩甲乙醛等；挥发性溶剂有乙醇、丙酮、乙酸乙酯或不同比例的混合溶剂等；增塑剂有甘油、丙二醇、山梨醇、邻苯二甲酸二甲酯和柠檬酸三乙酯等。

涂膜剂的工艺流程如图 3 – 13 所示。

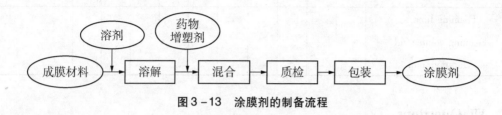

图 3 – 13　涂膜剂的制备流程

如果溶解成膜材料的溶剂也能溶解药物，可先将药物溶于溶剂中后加入；若不能直接溶解，则用少量溶剂将药物研细后加入。中药既可以提取液的方式加入，也可以直接将药物细粉分散到成膜材料溶液中。

涂膜剂可根据需要加入抑菌剂或抗氧剂。涂膜剂用于烧伤治疗，如果为非无菌制剂的，应在标签上标明"非无菌制剂"；产品说明书中应注明"本品为非无菌制剂"，同时在适应证下应明确标注"用于程度较轻的烧伤（Ⅰ度或浅Ⅱ度）"。涂膜剂质量检查项目有装量、无菌检查、微生物限度等。

三、预习思考

（1）理想的成膜材料应符合哪些要求？

（2）涂膜剂的优点与缺点有哪些？涂膜剂适用于什么状态的皮肤表面？

（3）涂膜剂可以用于哪些领域？

四、实验材料与仪器

1. 实验试剂与试药

聚乙烯醇 PVA（17 – 88）[①]、乙基纤维素（EC）、甘油、柠檬酸三乙酯、无水乙醇、蒸馏水、液体创面保护膜（哈尔滨乾佰纳生物药业有限公司）、雪山金罗汉止痛涂膜剂（西藏诺迪康药业股份有限公司）等。

2. 实验仪器

恒温水浴锅、鼓风烘箱、天平、培养皿、烧杯、游标卡尺等。

---

① "17"表示聚合度为 1 700～1 800，"88"表示醇解度均为 88%±2%。

五、实验内容

（一）PVA 涂膜剂
1. 处方

	处方 1
聚乙烯醇 PVA（17-88）	1.5 g
甘油	0.8 g
乙醇	10.0 g
蒸馏水	适量

2. 实验步骤

取处方量聚乙烯醇 PVA（17-88）于烧杯中，加约 10 mL 水浸泡 24 h 充分溶胀，于 95 ℃水浴加热至完全溶解，得 PVA 水溶液。搅拌下，将甘油、乙醇缓慢加入 PVA 溶液中，搅拌均匀，即得涂膜剂处方 1。

（二）*EC* 涂膜剂
1. 处方

	处方 2	处方 3
乙基纤维素	1.0 g	1.0 g
柠檬酸三乙酯	—	0.5 g
乙醇	适量	适量

2. 实验步骤

取 2.0 g 乙基纤维素（EC）于烧杯中，加约 20 mL 乙醇浸泡 24 h 充分溶胀，于 95 ℃水浴加热至完全溶解，得 10%（*W/V*）EC 乙醇溶液，即得涂膜剂处方 2。

将柠檬酸三乙酯缓慢加入 10ml 的 10%（*W/V*）EC 乙醇溶液中，搅拌均匀，即得涂膜剂处方 3。

注意事项

（1）成膜材料聚乙烯醇为亲水性高分子，其在水中的溶解须经历有限溶胀和无限溶胀两个过程。

（2）有限溶胀过程可将聚乙烯醇撒在水面静置，使水分子进入高分子内部，直至高分子空隙间充满水分子。有限溶胀必须充分，且温度不宜超过 40 ℃，以保证充分溶胀、溶解。由于经时较长，故须提前准备。

（3）随后进入无限溶胀过程，加热和/或搅拌可加速此过程。聚乙烯醇加热温度以 80～95 ℃为宜，温度过高可影响膜的溶解度和澄明度，并使膜的脆性增加。在加热过程中应避免溶剂挥发，以免影响实验结果。

六、实验结果与讨论

观察涂膜剂成膜外观，其应该完整光洁、厚度均一、色泽均匀、无明显气泡。同时，对涂膜剂的成膜时间、成膜性、成膜质地、柔韧性和撕拉完整性进行评价。

1. 皮肤测试

将制备的涂膜剂与液体创面保护膜（PVA 涂膜剂）及雪山金罗汉止痛涂膜剂（EC 涂膜剂）进行对比。

取涂膜剂少量（5～6 滴），涂抹于手臂内侧，形成厚度均一、直径为 2～3 cm 的近圆形区域（一式三份），观察膜的形成，记录成膜时间（表 3-47）。尝试将膜从皮肤撕下，观察膜的完整性。

表 3-47　涂膜剂在皮肤上的成膜时间

单位：min

编号	处方 1	处方 2	处方 3	市售制剂 1	市售制剂 2
1					
2					
3					
平均成膜时间（Mean ± SD）					
完整性					

2. 成膜性和成膜质地

取涂膜剂少量（约 1.5 g），轻轻地涂抹在玻璃培养皿底部，使其尽量形成厚度均一、直径为 5～6 cm 的近圆形区域。将培养皿置于 37 ℃鼓风烘箱中加热，观察成膜性（由液体或半固体转变成固体）。其间可用玻璃棒轻触涂膜剂表面，若无肉眼可见形变，证明涂膜剂已干燥成膜。

起膜前，观察已干燥的膜中是否有气泡，记录气泡数量。起膜过程中，观察涂膜剂是否有分层如固液分层或黏附于玻璃皿上。起膜后，用游标卡尺测量涂膜剂成膜后不同位置膜的厚度，评价厚度的均一性。将结果填入表 3-48 中。

表 3-48　涂膜剂的成膜性

	处方 1	处方 2	处方 3
是否分层			
气泡数量（个）			
成膜厚度/mm			

3. 柔韧性

起膜后将膜修剪成 0.5 cm × 1 cm 的矩形，固定矩形短边后轻轻拉伸，记录涂膜剂断裂前所能延展的最大长度，计算其断裂伸长率（表 3 – 49）。

表 3 – 49　涂膜剂的柔韧性

	处方 1	处方 2	处方 3
初始长度 L_0/cm			
最大延展长度 L/cm			
断裂伸长率 $[(L-L_0)/L_0]$ /%			

七、思考题

（1）常见的天然成膜材料有哪些，有哪些优点与不足？

（2）涂膜剂中常用的辅料有哪些，它们各起什么作用？

Experiment 12　Preparation of Pigments

I . Purpose

(1) To master the preparation of a small amount of pigments.

(2) Be familiar with the property and characteristics of commonly used film-forming materials.

(3) To have a general understanding of the quality inspections of pigments.

II . Principles

Pigments are liquid preparations in which active ingredients are dissolved or dispersed in solvent containing film-forming materials intended for external use on the affected area to form a film. The film, usually formed after solvent evaporation from pigments, will protect the affected area, and then the drug gradually released therefrom comes into its therapeutic effects. It is generally used for skin surface without exudation.

Pigments are usually composed of drugs, film-forming materials, volatile solvent, and plasticizers. Film-forming materials commonly used include polyvinyl alcohol, polyvinylpyrrolidone, ethyl cellulose and polyvinyl acetal; the volatile solvents are ethanol, acetone, ethyl acetate or solvents mixed with different volatile solvents in different proportions; plasticizers consist of glycerin, propylene glycol, sorbitol, dimethyl phthalate and triethyl citrate. The process flow of the pigments is detailed in figure 3 – 13.

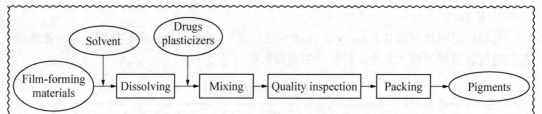

Figure 3 –13　Flow chart of the preparation of pigments

　　If the drug is soluble in the solvent in which film-forming materials dissolved, the drug can be dissolved in the solvent firstly before addition; if not, just add the drug to the solvent and grind to uniform before addition. The traditional Chinese medicine can be directly added in the form of extract or dispersing powders into the solvent before addition.

　　The pigments may include disinfectants or antioxidants if necessary. If the pigments are used for burn treatment but non-sterile preparation, they should be marked as "non-sterile preparation" on the label as well as in the product specification. What's more, the notice of "for less severe burns (I degree or light II degree)" should be clearly indicated in the indications. The quality inspection of pigments includes filling, sterility and microbial limit.

III. Preview

　　(1) What are the requirements for an ideal film-forming material?

　　(2) What are the advantages and disadvantages of pigments? What are the clinical indications?

　　(3) Which fields can pigments be used for?

IV. Experimental materials and equipments

　　1. Reagents and experimental materials

　　Polyvinyl alcohol PVA (17 – 88), ethyl cellulose (EC), glycerin, triethyl citrate, anhydrous ethanol, distilled water, Cuts Waterproof Pigmeng (Qian Benefiting Biopharma, Harbin), Jokul Golden Arhat Acesodyne Liniment (Tibet Rhodiola Pharmaceutical Holding Co. , Xizang).

　　2. Experimental equipments

　　Constant temperature water bath, blowing heat chambers, balance, culture dish, beaker and vernier caliper.

V. Experiment content

　　1. Preparation of PVA pigments

　　(1) Formulation:

	Formular 1
Polyvinyl alcohol PVA (17 – 88)	1.5 g
Glycerin	0.8 g
Ethanol	10.0 g
Distilled water	q. s

(2) Procedures:

Put polyvinyl alcohol PVA (17 – 88) in a beaker, add 15 mL of water and make it soaked for 24 h until swelling. And incubate it in a constant temperature water bath at 95 ℃ until it completely dissolves to obtain PVA aqueous solution. Under stirring, slowly add glycerin and ethanol to the PVA solution and stir evenly to obtain pigments formulation 1.

2. Preparation of EC pigments

(1) Formulation:

	Formular 2	Formular 3
Ethyl cellulose	1.0 g	1.0 g
Triethyl citrate	–	0.5 g
Ethanol	q. s	q. s

(2) Procedures:

Weigh ethyl cellulose (EC) 2.0 g in a beaker, add appropriate 20mL of ethanol and make it soaked for 24 h until swelling. And incubate it in a constant temperature water bath at 95 ℃ until it completely dissolves to obtain 10% (W/V) EC ethanol solution, that is pigments formulation 2.

Slowly add triethyl citrate into 10 mL of 10% (W/V) EC ethanol solution and stir evenly to obtain pigments formulation 3.

[Precautions]

(1) The film-forming material, polyvinyl alcohol, is a kind of hydrophilic polymer. Its dissolution in water generally undergoes two processes, that is, limited swelling and unlimited swelling.

(2) For the limited swelling, polyvinyl alcohol could be sprinkled on the surface of the water, allowing its interior to be immersed by water molecules until the polymer pores are filled fully with water molecules. The process of limited swelling shall be conducted sufficiently at a temperature lower than 40 ℃ to ensure adequate swelling and dissolution. This process takes time and should be prepared in advance.

(3) Following the limited swelling process is the unlimited swelling process, which can be accelerated by heating or/and stirring. The appropriate heating temperature for polyvinyl alcohol is preferably 80 ~ 95 ℃. The excessive temperature may decrease the solubility and clarity of

the film and increase the brittleness of the film. Solvent loss should be avoided during heating.

VI. Experiment results and discussion

Observe the appearance of films, which should be holonomic and smooth, uniform in thickness and color without obvious bubbles after the pigments form films. Meanwhile, evaluate film-forming time, film formability, film texture, film flexibility and tear integrity of the films.

1. Skin test

Compare the prepared pigments with Cuts Waterproof Pigmeng (PVA pigments) and Jokul Golden Arhat Acesodyne Liniment (EC pigments).

Spread the pigments (5～6 drops) to the interior side of the armto form approximate circular regions with a diameter 2～3 cm (triplicate). Observe the formation of films, and record the film-forming time (Table 3－47). Try to remove the films from the skin and observe the integrity of the films.

Table 3－47　Film forming time of pigments on the skin   Unit：min

Number	Formulation 1	Formulation 2	Formulation 3	Commercial preparation 1	Commercial preparation 2
1					
2					
3					
Average film-forming time (*Mean ± SD*)					
Integrality					

2. Film formability and film texture

A small amount of the pigments (about 1.5 g) were gently spread on the bottom of glass culture dish to form approximate circular regions with a diameter about 5～6 cm. Place the dish in a blowing heat chambers at 37 ℃, observe film-forming time (i. e., converting from liquid, then semi-solid to solid). If there is no obvious deformation when wiping the surface of films with a glass rob, the films are successfully prepared.

Before the film is uncovered, observe whether there are bubbles in the dried film, count the number of bubbles. When uncovering the films, observe whether there is delamination such as solid-liquid layering or adhesion to the glass dish. In order to evaluate the uniformity, the thickness of the uncovered film was measured by vernier caliper at different positions. Fill the result in Table 3－48.

Table 3 −48 Film formability of Pigments

	Formulation 1	Formulation 2	Formulation 3
Delamination or not			
Number of bubbles			
Thickness /mm			

3. Flexibility

Cut the formed film to a rectangle of 0. 5 cm × 1 cm, and gently stretched the film by the short side of the rectangle. Record the maximum length that pigments can be extended before broken and calculate elongation at break (Table 3 −49).

Table 3 −49 Flexibility of Solution Type Pigments

	Formulation 1	Formulation 2	Formulation 3
Initial length L_0/cm			
Maximum extended length L /cm			
Elongation at break $[(L-L_0)/L_0]/\%$			

VII. Questions

(1) What are the common natural film-forming materials? What are their advantages and disadvantages?

(2) What are the commonly used excipients of pigments? What roles do they play?

第四部分　新剂型与新技术

实验一　固体分散体的制备与验证

一、实验目的

(1) 掌握熔融法和溶剂法制备固体分散体。
(2) 熟悉固体分散体的鉴定方法。
(3) 了解热熔挤出技术制备固体分散体。

二、实验原理

固体分散体 (solid dispersion) 系指药物以分子、无定形或微晶等状态均匀分散在固态载体中所形成的分散体系。固体分散体的主要特点是利用不同性质的载体使药物高度分散以满足不同用药目的，如提高难溶性药物的溶解度和溶出速率，缓释药物或控制药物在小肠释放等。固体分散体作为中间产物，可根据需要进一步制成胶囊剂、片剂、软膏剂、栓剂以及注射剂等。

固体分散体的载体材料可分为水溶性、难溶性和肠溶性材料三大类。在选用载体材料时可根据制备目的选择单一或混合载体。常见的水溶性载体材料有聚乙二醇类、聚维酮类等；难溶性载体材料有乙基纤维素、聚丙烯酸树脂等；肠溶性载体材料有纤维素类、肠溶型聚丙烯酸树脂等。

固体分散体制备方法主要有：①熔融法。熔融法是指将药物与载体混匀，加热至熔融，熔融物在搅拌下迅速冷却成固体。该方法适用于对温度稳定的药物，以及熔点低或者不溶于有机溶剂的载体材料。不耐热的药物与载体不适合本法。②溶剂法（共沉淀法）。溶剂法是指将药物与载体材料共同溶解于有机溶剂中，蒸发除去有机溶剂后使药物与载体材料同时析出。该方法适用于熔点较高或热敏感性的药物和载体。③溶剂熔融法：溶剂熔融法是指将药物用适当的溶剂溶解，与熔融载体混合均匀后，蒸发除去有机溶剂，迅速冷却固化后得到固体分散体。该法是熔融和溶剂法的联合应用，适于高熔点对热敏感药物，也适用于液体药物。④热熔挤出法：热熔挤出法是指将药物和载体预先混合后，置于逐段加热的热熔挤出机中，通过加热和剪切作用，将药物和辅料熔融混合，使药物高度分散在固体载体材料中。热熔挤出法具有无须有机溶剂、生产效率高、适用于工业化生产等优势。

固体分散体的物相鉴别方法有差示扫描量热分析法、粉末 X 射线衍射法、红外光谱法、核磁共振法等，必要时可同时采用几种方法进行鉴别。

三、预习思考

（1）查找列举 1～2 种采用固体分散体技术制备的市售制剂，结合药物性质阐述其制备成固体分散体的目的。

（2）预习实验内容，明确处方中药物与各种辅料的性质及用途。

（3）了解差示扫描量热分析及粉末 X 射线衍射鉴定固体分散体物相的原理。

四、实验材料与仪器

1. 实验试剂与试药

布洛芬、交联聚乙烯吡咯烷酮（Kollidon® CL-F）、聚乙烯吡咯烷酮 K-30（PVP K-30）、羟丙基甲基纤维素（HPMC E5）、聚乙烯吡咯烷酮 VA64（PVP VA64）、聚乙烯己内酰胺 - 聚乙酸乙烯酯 - 聚乙二醇接枝共聚物（Soluplus®）、无水乙醇、甲醇。

2. 实验仪器

天平、蒸发皿、研钵、表面皿、量筒、烧杯、电加热套、容量瓶、注射器、微孔滤膜、恒温水浴锅、真空干燥箱、热熔挤出机、紫外分光光度计、溶出试验仪、差示扫描量热仪、粉末 X 射线衍射仪。

五、实验内容

（一）布洛芬固体分散体的制备（熔融法）

1. 处方

布洛芬	2.0 g
Kollidon® CL-F	10.0 g

2. 实验步骤

采用熔融法，布洛芬与 Kollidon® CL-F 分别粉碎过 60 目筛，取处方量药物及载体混合均匀，置蒸发皿内，100 ℃电热套加热熔融后恒温搅拌 30 min。迅速倒入预冷的表面皿中，用塑料薄膜包裹，置于冰浴至表面完全固化，在 - 20 ℃冰箱中冷冻 30 min。

除去包裹的塑料薄膜，置真空干燥箱中 40 ℃ 干燥 24 h。取出，用研钵研细，粉碎过 60 目筛，即得布洛芬固体分散体。

按处方比例称取粉碎过 60 目筛的载体与药物混合均匀，再次过 60 目筛，制备得到物理混合物，作为实验对照组。

3. 质量评价

1）溶出速率测定。取布洛芬 100 mg、相当于 100 mg 布洛芬的固体分散体及其同比例物理混合物，精密称定，备用。

（1）标准曲线的绘制。精密称取干燥至恒重的布洛芬 20 mg，置于 100 mL 容量瓶中，加甲醇溶解、定容，摇匀，作为储备液。分别精密吸取上述储备液 0.25 mL、0.50 mL、1.00 mL、2.50 mL 和 5.00 mL 于 10 mL 容量瓶中，加水定容，摇匀，以水为空白对照，在 263 nm 处测定吸光度。以吸光度值对布洛芬浓度作线性回归，得布洛芬标准曲线方程。

（2）溶出度测定。按照溶出度与释放度测定法（2020 版《中国药典》通则 0931 第二法）进行。具体操作参照附录 II，溶出介质为 900 mL 蒸馏水，转速为 100 r/min，温度（37 ± 0.5）℃。

取经超声脱气的溶出介质 900 mL 置于溶出杯中，待杯内温度恒定（37 ± 0.5）℃，取样品投入溶出杯，分别于 5 min、10 min、15 min、30 min、45 min、60 min、90 min 和 120 min 吸取溶出介质 5 mL（补加等体积相同温度的溶出介质），经 0.45 μm 微孔滤膜过滤。续滤液在 263 nm 处测定吸光度，每种样品平行 3 份。按标准曲线方程，计算不同时间累积溶出百分率，绘制溶出曲线，比较各样品的溶出度行为。

2）物相鉴别。差示扫描量热分析（differential scanning calorimetry，DSC）用来检验固体分散体中是否存在药物晶体。若存在药物结晶，则有熔点吸热峰存在；药物晶体存在越多，吸热峰总面积越大。取布洛芬、布洛芬固体分散体及其同比例物理混合物置于 DSC 铝坩埚中（约 5 mg），以空白铝坩埚为参比。DSC 工作条件为：氮气气氛，升温速率 10 ℃/min，温度扫描范围 30 ～ 150 ℃，绘制 DSC 曲线。

粉末 X 射线衍射法（powder X-ray diffractometry，PXRD）研究的对象是有众多取向的随机小晶体的总和。利用该方法所测得的每种晶体的衍射强度和分布都有特殊规律，可获得晶形变化的信息，据此可以定性分析固体分散体中药物的存在状态。分别对布洛芬、布洛芬固体分散体及其同比例物理混合物进行 X 射线衍射分析。分析条件为：Cu-Kα辐射；管流 20 mA；高压强度 40 kV；扫描范围（2θ）：5°～ 45°；步长：0.05°；扫描速率：5°/min。

（二）布洛芬固体分散体的制备（溶剂法）

1. 处方

布洛芬	0.5 g
PVP K-30	2.5 g

2. 实验步骤

采用溶剂法，取布洛芬 0.5 g 置于蒸发皿内，加入无水乙醇 10 mL，在 50 ～ 60 ℃ 水浴上加热溶解。加入 PVP K-30 2.5 g，搅拌溶解后将水浴温度提高至 80 ～ 90 ℃，继续搅拌并充分蒸去溶剂。取下蒸发皿，样品于 40 ℃真空干燥 2 ～ 3 h，粉碎过 60 目筛，即得布洛芬固体分散体。

按处方比例称取粉碎过 60 目筛的 PVP K-30 与布洛芬，混合均匀后再次过 60 目筛，制备得到物理混合物，作为实验对照组。

3. 质量评价

参照"五、（一）3."项的操作。

（三）布洛芬固体分散体的制备（热熔挤出法）

1. 处方

热熔挤出法制备布洛芬固体分散体的处方组成见表 4 - 1。

表 4 - 1　热熔挤出法制备布洛芬固体分散体的处方组成

处方编号	药物 布洛芬/g	载体			药物比例/%
		HPMC E5/g	PVP VA64/g	Soluplus®/g	
H1	3.0	27.0	—	—	10
H2	6.0	24.0	—	—	20
H3	12.0	18.0	—	—	40
P1	3.0	—	27.0	—	10
P2	6.0	—	24.0	—	20
P3	12.0	—	18.0	—	40
S1	3.0	—	—	27.0	10
S2	6.0	—	—	24.0	20
S3	12.0	—	—	18.0	40

2. 实验步骤

按各处方准确称取布洛芬和载体，在研钵中充分混匀。待热熔挤出机的温度及螺杆转速平衡后，将混合物加至双螺杆挤出机。挤出温度为 170 ℃，转速为 100 r/min，记录扭矩。挤出物室温放置冷却后，粉碎过 60 目筛，在干燥器中保存。

3. 质量评价

参照"五、（一）3."项的操作。

4. 布洛芬固体分散体的处方筛选

根据上述各处方布洛芬固体分散体的溶出实验与物相鉴别结果，综合评价载药量和载体材料种类对固体分散体中药物分散效果的影响。

注意事项

（1）熔融法制备固体分散体时，为避免湿气的引入，建议采用酒精灯或者天然气火源，在石棉网上加热，或者用电炉或电热套进行加热。

（2）熔融法制备固体分散体时，搅拌速度不宜过快，防止引入空气。

（3）熔融法制备固体分散体时，搅拌时间过短可能导致药物分散不匀。

（4）溶剂法制备固体分散体时，溶剂蒸发速度是影响药物结晶析出的重要因素。溶剂蒸发速度过快，药物分子聚集时间不足，结晶析出减少。

（5）溶剂法中溶解与蒸发两个过程均可用旋转蒸发仪完成。

六、实验结果与讨论

（一）布洛芬固体分散体的制备（熔融法）

1. 布洛芬标准曲线

以布洛芬浓度为横坐标，吸光度值 A 为纵坐标，绘制布洛芬标准曲线。

2. 溶出度测定结果

将熔融法制备布洛芬固体分散体溶出测定结果填入表 4-2。

表 4-2　熔融法制备布洛芬固体分散体溶出测定结果

时间/min	累积溶出率平均值/%		
	布洛芬	布洛芬物理混合物	布洛芬固体分散体
5			
10			
15			
30			
45			
60			
90			
120			

3. 绘制溶出曲线

以取样时间 t 为横坐标，布洛芬累积溶出率（%）为纵坐标，绘制实验样品的溶出曲线，比较固体分散体与原料药、物理混合物的溶出度差异。

（二）布洛芬固体分散体的制备（溶剂法）

1. 溶出度测定结果

将溶剂法制备布洛芬固体分散体溶出测定结果填入表 4-3。

表 4-3　溶剂法制备布洛芬固体分散体溶出测定结果

时间/min	累积溶出率平均值/%		
	布洛芬	布洛芬物理混合物	布洛芬固体分散体
5			

续表4-3

时间/min	累积溶出率平均值/%		
	布洛芬	布洛芬物理混合物	布洛芬固体分散体
10			
15			
30			
45			
60			
90			
120			

2. 绘制溶出曲线

以取样时间 t 为横坐标，布洛芬累积溶出率（%）为纵坐标，绘制实验样品的溶出曲线，比较固体分散体与原料药、物理混合物的溶出度差异。

（三）布洛芬固体分散体的制备（热熔挤出法）

1. 溶出度测定结果

将溶出度测定结果填入表4-4。

表4-4 热熔挤出法制备布洛芬固体分散体溶出测定结果

处方编号	累积溶出率平均值/%							
	5 min	10 min	15 min	30 min	45 min	60 min	90 min	120 min
H1								
H2								
H3								
P1								
P2								
P3								
S1								
S2								
S3								

2. 绘制溶出曲线

以取样时间 t 为横坐标，布洛芬累积溶出率（%）为纵坐标，绘制不同载体不同药物比例的布洛芬溶出曲线。

七、思考题

（1）固体分散体在贮藏期内容易发生老化现象，如何延缓其老化并提高稳定性？

（2）简述固体分散体提高难溶性药物溶出度的原理。

（3）除制成固体分散体外，还有哪些方法可以增加难溶性固体药物的溶解度或溶出速度？

（4）简述固体分散体载体材料选择的主要依据。

参考文献

［1］徐璐. 基于改善布洛芬溶出行为的固体分散体制备方法与性质评价［D］.沈阳：沈阳药科大学，2009.

［2］魏敏. 三种方法制备的布洛芬固体分散体及其性质比较［D］.沈阳：沈阳药科大学，2009.

［3］董品. 共混聚合物抑制热熔挤出无定形固体分散体双重结晶的研究［D］.广州：中山大学，2015.

实验二　　包合物的制备与验证

一、实验目的

（1）掌握包合物的制备方法。

（2）掌握包合率及载药量的计算方法。

（3）熟悉包合物的验证方法。

（4）熟悉 β - 环糊精及其衍生物的性质和应用。

二、实验原理

包合物（inclusion compound）系指一种分子被包嵌于另一种分子的空穴结构内形成的分子囊（molecular capsules），亦称分子包衣。由主分子及客分子两部分组成，主分子一般具有较大空穴结构，足以将客分子容纳在内，形成分子微囊。药物制成包合物后可增加药物的溶解度，提高药物的口服生物利用度，使液态药物粉末化，此外还可防止挥发性成分挥发，掩盖药物不良气味或味道，调节药物的释放速率，提高药物稳定性和降低药物毒副反应等。

药物制剂中常用的包合材料为环糊精（cyclodextrin，CD），常见的 CD 有 α、β、γ 3 种，分别由 6、7、8 个葡萄糖分子通过 α－1，4－糖苷键连接而成。三种环糊精的空穴内径与物理性质存在较大差异。其中，β－环糊精（β-CD）的空穴内径为 0.7～0.8 nm，25 ℃水中溶解度为 18.5 g/L，随着温度升高溶解度增大，在 40 ℃、60 ℃、80 ℃ 和 100 ℃时的溶解度分别为 37 g/L、80 g/L、183 g/L 和 256 g/L。将 β-CD 部分羟基上的氢原子用羟丙基取代，可以得到水溶性高的羟丙基－β－环糊精（HP-β-CD）。

包合物的制备方法有饱和水溶液法、研磨法、超声法、冷冻干燥法、喷雾干燥法等。其中以饱和水溶液法最为常用，即用主分子的饱和溶液与客分子相混，使客分子进入主分子的空穴中，用适当的方式（如冷藏、浓缩、加沉淀剂等）使包合物析出，再将得到的固体包合物过滤、洗涤、干燥。

包合是物理过程而不是化学反应，包合物能否形成且稳定存在主要取决于环糊精和药物的空间结构及极性。药物必须与环糊精的空穴形状和大小相适应才能够稳定存在。另外，包合物的形成和稳定性也与客分子的极性有关。包合物中主分子和客分子的比例一般为非化学计量，因为主分子的空穴仅部分可以被客分子占据，空穴数仅决定客分子的最大填入量，只要客分子不超过最大填入量，主、客分子数之比可以在一定范围内变化。

包合物的验证主要是鉴别药物与环糊精是否形成了包合物。目前常用的验证方法有相溶解度法、薄层色谱法、热分析法、X 射线衍射法、红外光谱法等。

三、预习思考

（1）简述包合物中常用环糊精的种类、性质及各自的特点。
（2）包合物的常用制备方法有哪些？
（3）根据薄荷油的性质和用途，思考将其制成包合物的目的。
（4）简述薄层色谱法鉴别包合物的基本原理与步骤。

四、实验材料与仪器

1. 实验试剂与试药

薄荷油、柚皮素、β－环糊精、羟丙基－β－环糊精（HP-β-CD，分子量为 1 402）、无水乙醇、石油醚、乙酸乙酯、香荚兰醛、浓硫酸、蒸馏水。

2. 实验仪器

100 mL 具塞锥形瓶、硅胶 G 板、TLC 展开槽、量筒、容量瓶、天平、恒温水浴锅、控温磁力搅拌器、玻璃棒、抽滤装置、0.45 μm 微孔滤膜、真空干燥箱、差示扫描量热仪、紫外－可见分光光度计、80 目筛。

五、实验内容

（一）薄荷油–β–环糊精包合物的制备（饱和水溶液法）

1. 处方

薄荷油	1 mL（0.908 g）
β–环糊精	4 g
蒸馏水	50 mL

2. 实验步骤

称取 β–环糊精 4 g，置于 100 mL 具塞锥形瓶中，加水 50 mL，加热溶解，（50±1）℃ 保温，备用。

精密称取薄荷油 0.908 g 或量取 1 mL，在磁力搅拌下缓缓滴入上述（50±1）℃ 保温的 β–环糊精水溶液中，恒温搅拌 2.5 h，冰箱冷藏放置，待沉淀完全析出后抽滤，用无水乙醇洗涤 3 次至沉淀表面无油渍，置真空干燥器中干燥，即得。

3. 质量评价

1）性状：评价包合物的色泽、气味等。

2）物相鉴定。

（1）薄层色谱分析（thin-layer chromatography，TLC）。取薄荷油 1 滴加入 1 mL 95% 乙醇中摇匀，得薄荷油溶液；取 β–环糊精适量，加入 1 mL 95% 乙醇溶液中摇匀，得 β–环糊精溶液；称取薄荷油–β–环糊精包合物 0.3 g，加 95% 乙醇溶液 2 mL 振摇，过滤，得包合物溶液；另取薄荷油和 β–环糊精物理混合物，同法制备物理混合物溶液。取以上四种溶液各约 10 μL，分别点于同一硅胶 G 板上，以石油醚–乙酸乙酯（17∶3）为展开剂展开，用 5% 香荚兰醛浓硫酸溶液为显色剂，烘干显色。

（2）差示扫描量热分析（DSC）。取薄荷油、包合物、物理混合物和 β–环糊精各 5 mg 置于 DSC 铝坩埚中，以空白铝坩埚为参比，设置 DSC 工作条件为：氮气气氛，升温速率 10 ℃/min，温度扫描范围 30～340 ℃。

（二）柚皮素–羟丙基–β–环糊精（HP-β-CD）包合物的制备

1. 处方

柚皮素	0.4 g
HP-β-CD	2.0 g
蒸馏水	50 mL

2. 实验步骤

称取 HP-β-CD 2.0 g，置于 100 mL 具塞锥形瓶中，加水 50 mL，加热溶解，(40±1) ℃ 保温，备用。

称取柚皮素 0.4 g，加无水乙醇 5 mL，超声使完全溶解，在磁力搅拌下加入于 40 ℃ 保温的 HP-β-CD 的溶液质量中（此时柚皮素与 HP-β-CD 摩尔比为 1∶1），搅拌 12 h，放至室温，经 0.45 μm 微孔滤膜过滤，将滤液于 40 ℃ 真空干燥，过 80 目筛，即得。

3. 质量评价

（1）物相鉴定。差示扫描量热分析（DSC）：取柚皮素、包合物、物理混合物及 HP-β-CD 各 5 mg，置 DSC 铝坩埚中，以空白铝坩埚为参比，设置 DSC 工作条件为：氮气气流，升温速率 10 ℃/min，温度范围 30～300 ℃。

（2）包合率与载药量的测定。标准曲线的测定：精密称取柚皮素 16 mg 置于 100 mL 容量瓶中，用乙醇溶解并定容至刻度。分别精密量取 1.0 mL、1.5 mL、2.0 mL、2.5 mL 和 3.0 mL 上述溶液至 50 mL 容量瓶中，用乙醇定容至刻度，摇匀（浓度为 3.2～9.6 μg/mL）。在 288 nm 处测定溶液的吸光度。以柚皮素浓度对吸光度进行线性回归，得标准曲线方程。

包合率与载药量的测定：精密称取包合物 15 mg 于 25 mL 容量瓶中，加乙醇溶解并定容，稀释适当倍数后在 288 nm 波长处测定吸光度，根据标准曲线计算包合物中柚皮素含量。包合率（inclusion rate）和载药量（drug loading，以 DL 表示）计算公式为式（4-2-1）及式（4-2-2）：

$$包合率 = \frac{M_1}{M_2} \times 100\% \tag{4-2-1}$$

$$DL = \frac{M_1}{M_3} \times 100\% \tag{4-2-2}$$

式中，M_1 表示包合物中药物质量，M_2 表示总投药量，M_3 表示包合物总质量。

4. 包合物处方工艺影响因素考察

探究不同处方、工艺对柚皮素-HP-β-CD 包合物包合率和载药量的影响。

（1）乙醇与水的体积比。固定柚皮素与 HP-β-CD 的摩尔质量比为 1∶1，在 40 ℃ 磁力搅拌 12 h 制备包合物，考察乙醇与水体积比分别为 2∶1、1∶1、1∶2 和 1∶6 对包合物包合率和载药量的影响。

（2）搅拌时间。固定柚皮素与 HP-β-CD 的摩尔质量比为 1∶1，乙醇与水体积比为 1∶1，在 40 ℃ 分别磁力搅拌 4 h、8 h、12 h 和 24 h，考察搅拌时间对包合率和载药量的影响。

（3）包合温度。固定柚皮素与 HP-β-CD 的摩尔质量比为 1∶1，乙醇与水体积比为 1∶1，分别在 40 ℃、60 ℃ 和 80 ℃ 下以磁力搅拌 12 h 制备包合物，考察包合温度对包合率和载药量的影响。

注意事项

（1）β-CD 包合物的制备温度为（50 ± 1）℃，制备过程搅拌时间要充分且须在密闭容器中进行，以防止薄荷油挥发。最后用无水乙醇洗涤时应避免过度洗涤，否则影响包合率。

（2）柚皮素水溶性差，需用适量有机溶剂将其溶解才能够保证其在包合反应过程中处于分子状态，从而有利于它进入 HP-β-CD 空腔内，但是有机溶剂对已经形成的包合物有一定的解包合作用，并且可能与药物分子竞争主分子，因此选择适当的醇/水十分重要。

六、实验结果与讨论

（一）薄荷油 – β-CD 包合物的制备

（1）观察薄荷油 – β-CD 的外观性状。

（2）包合物物相鉴定。①绘制（拍摄）TLC 图，比较包合物和物理混合物中薄荷油的特征斑点以及 R_f 值，并分析原因。②绘制 DSC 图，比较包合物与物理混合物的 DSC 结果差异，并分析原因。

（二）柚皮素 – HP-β-CD 包合物的制备

1. 包合物物相鉴定

绘制 DSC 图，比较包合物与物理混合物的 DSC 结果差异，并分析原因。

2. 包合率与载药量测定

（1）柚皮素标准曲线。以柚皮素浓度为横坐标，吸光度 A 为纵坐标，绘制柚皮素标准曲线。

（2）包合率与载药量计算。根据标准曲线计算包合物中柚皮素含量，计算包合物的包合率和载药量。

3. 包合物处方工艺对包合物包合率与载药量的影响

（1）乙醇与水的体积比（表 4 – 5）。

表 4 – 5　醇/水对包合率和载药量的影响

醇/水（V/V）	包合率/%	载药量/%
2 : 1		
1 : 1		
1 : 2		
1 : 6		

（2）搅拌时间（表4-6）。

表4-6　搅拌时间对包合率和载药量的影响

搅拌时间/h	包合率/%	载药量/%
4		
8		
12		
24		

（3）包合温度（表4-7）。

表4-7　包合温度对包合率和载药量的影响

温度/℃	包合率/%	载药量/%
40		
60		
80		

七、思考题

（1）β-环糊精的包合物通常采用饱和溶液法制备，而 HP-β-CD 的包合试验却采用溶液搅拌法，结合两种环糊精的性质分析其原因。

（2）结合影响因素考察结果，思考乙醇与水的体积比、搅拌时间及包合温度等因素对包合物的载药量和包合率产生影响的可能原因。

（3）除了 TLC 与 DSC 法，还有哪些方法可以用于包合物形成的鉴定？简述其鉴定原理。

（4）查找已上市的包合物制剂，说明包合物提高药物口服生物利用度的原理。

参考文献

[1] 崔福德. 药剂学实验指导 [M].2 版. 北京：人民卫生出版社，2007.

[2] 解春英. 羟丙基-β-环糊精包合对柚皮素增溶作用研究 [D].浙江：浙江大学，2011.

[3] 国家药典委员会. 中华人民共和国药典 [M].北京：中国医药科技出版社，2020.

实验三　微球的制备及评价

一、实验目的

(1) 掌握乳化 – 溶剂挥发法（液中干燥法）制备微球。
(2) 熟悉制备微球的常用辅料。
(3) 熟悉微球的质量检查方法。
(4) 了解制备微球的新方法。

二、实验原理

微球（microspheres）系指药物溶解或分散在载体辅料中形成的微小球状实体。通常粒径在 $1 \sim 250\ \mu m$ 之间，一般制成混悬剂供注射或口服。药物制成微球后通常具备以下特点：一定的靶向作用；缓释或控释性能；更好的稳定性。

微球的载体材料可分为三类：天然高分子材料，如明胶、壳聚糖、海藻酸盐、蛋白质等；半合成高分子材料，多为纤维素衍生物，如乙基纤维素、甲基纤维素、羟丙基纤维素等；合成高分子材料，常用的有聚乳酸（polylactic acid，PLA）和聚乳酸 – 羟基乙酸共聚物（poly lactic-co-glycolic acid，PLGA）等。

微球的常用制备方法包括乳化 – 溶剂挥发法（液中干燥法）、乳化 – 化学交联法、乳化 – 加热固化法、喷雾干燥法和旋碟法等。乳化 – 溶剂挥发法是将不相混溶的两相通过机械搅拌或超声乳化的方式制成乳剂，内相溶剂挥发除去，成球材料固化析出成微球，是最常用的微球制备方法。另外，超细微粒制备系统（ultra-fine particle processing system，UPPS）是一种新型微球制备方法，利用液体 – 气体界面张力作用维持液滴球形的原理，溶液经高速旋碟剪切雾化成微滴，悬浮在受控气流中，溶剂随气流运动快速蒸发后，药物与载体逐渐固化形成微球。

微球质量评价的指标包括形态、粒径及其分布、载药量、包封率和释放速度等。

三、预习思考

(1) 微球的常用制备方法有哪些？分别适用于什么种类的载体材料？
(2) 掌握粒径及粒径分布的表示方法。
(3) 掌握实验内容，明确处方中药物与辅料的用途。
(4) 了解超细微粒制备系统的基本结构和工作原理。

四、实验材料与仪器

1. 实验试剂与试药

石杉碱甲、聚乳酸－羟基乙酸共聚物（PLGA）、聚乙烯醇（PVA）、二氯甲烷、碳酸二甲酯、乙腈、浓盐酸、碳酸二氢钾、磷酸、去离子水。

2. 实验仪器

烧杯、量筒、天平、容量瓶、光学显微镜、扫描电子显微镜、高速离心机、冷冻干燥仪、高效液相色谱仪、超细微粒制备系统、磁力搅拌器、激光粒度分析仪、蠕动泵。

五、实验内容

（一）石杉碱甲 PLGA 微球的制备（乳化－溶剂挥发法）

1. 处方

石杉碱甲	0.10 g
PLGA	1.00 g

2. 实验步骤

采用 O/W 乳化－溶剂挥发法制备石杉碱甲 PLGA 微球。将 PLGA 和药物共同溶于 10 mL 二氯甲烷中形成油相。将 2.0 g PVA 溶于 100 mL 水中，形成水相。在机械搅拌下将油相加入水相中，进行乳化。10 min 后，降低搅拌速率，室温常压下让溶剂挥发。离心，去离子水洗涤后收集微球，冷冻干燥 48 h 即得。

3. 质量评价

（1）微球的外观形态。

采用光学显微镜、扫描电镜观察微球的外观形态。

（2）粒径及其分布。

根据《中国药典》2020 版 9014 微粒制剂指导原则，微粒制剂需提供粒径的平均值及其分布的数据或图形。采用动态光散射法（干法）测定微球的粒径。Malvern 2000 激光粒度分析仪参数设置参考值如下：分散气压为 1.5 bar，遮光度 0.5%～6.0%，测量时间 8～12 s，每个样品平行测定 3 次。

微粒制剂粒径分布数据，常用各粒径范围内的粒子数或百分率表示；有时也可用跨距表示，跨距愈小分布愈窄，即粒子大小愈均匀。

根据式（4-3-1）计算跨距（span，以 S 表示）：

$$S = \frac{(D_{90} - D_{10})}{D_{50}} \tag{4-3-1}$$

式中，D_{10}、D_{50}、D_{90} 分别指粒径累积分布图中 10%、50%、90% 处所对应的粒径。

以粒径为横坐标，以频率（每一粒径范围的粒子个数除以粒子总数所得的百分率）为纵坐标作图，即得粒径分布直方图；以各粒径范围的频率对各粒径范围的平均值作图，即得粒径分布曲线。

（3）载药量与包封率。

石杉碱甲标准曲线：精密称取干燥至恒重的石杉碱甲 25 mg，置于 50 mL 容量瓶中，用 0.01 mol/L 盐酸溶解并定容，得浓度为 500 μg/mL 的贮备液。精密量取贮备液适量，分别用 0.01 mol/L 盐酸稀释定容至浓度为 0.25 μg/mL、2.50 μg/mL、10.00 μg/mL、20.00 μg/mL、50.00 μg/mL，采用高效液相色谱法记录峰面积。以药物浓度对峰面积进行线性回归，得石杉碱甲标准曲线方程。

高效液相色谱条件：以十八烷基硅烷键合硅胶为填充剂；以磷酸盐缓冲液（取磷酸二氢钾 2.72 g，加水 1 000 mL 溶解，用磷酸调节 pH 至 2.5）－乙腈（86∶14）为流动相；检测波长为 310 nm；流速为 1.0 mL/min；进样量为 20 μL。

微球中药物含量测定：将精密称量的微球（约 10 mg）溶于盛有 1 mL 乙腈的 25 mL 容量瓶中，以 0.01 mol/L 的盐酸定容，沉淀聚合物。剧烈振摇容量瓶使聚合物沉淀完全，微孔滤膜过滤后测定溶液中石杉碱甲的含量。微球载药量（drug loading，以 DL 表示）和包封率（entrapment efficiency，以 EE 表示）的计算公式分别为式（4－3－2）和式（4－3－3）：

$$DL = \frac{M_1}{M_2} \times 100\% \qquad\qquad (4-3-2)$$

$$EE = \frac{M_1}{M_3} \times 100\% \qquad\qquad (4-3-3)$$

式中，M_1 表示微球中药物质量，M_2 表示微球总质量，M_3 表示投药量。

（4）微球处方因素考察。

水相中乳化剂的含量：当投药量石杉碱甲与 PLGA 的质量比为 1∶10，油相中 PLGA 的浓度为 10%，油与水的体积比为 1∶10，机械搅拌转速为 800 r/min 时，以 3 种不同浓度的 PVA 水溶液（1%，2%，3%）作为水相制备微球，分别测定微球的粒径及其分布、载药量、包封率等指标。

油相中聚合物的浓度：当投药量石杉碱甲与 PLGA 比例为 1∶10，水相中 PVA 浓度为 2%，油与水的体积比为 1∶10，机械搅拌转速为 800 r/min 时，以 3 种不同浓度的 PLGA 浓度（5%，10%，20%）制备微球，分别测定微球的粒径及其分布、载药量、包封率等指标。

（二）超细微粒制备系统制备 PLGA 微球

1. 处方

石杉碱甲	0.24 g
PLGA	2.40 g

2. 实验步骤

按处方称取 PLGA 固体颗粒，溶于 20 mL 二氯甲烷与 40 mL 碳酸二甲酯的混合溶剂中，加入处方量的药物，搅拌得到均匀的含药溶液。将所得溶液经蠕动泵供应至 UPPS 的圆碟中心，调节供液速率为 3 r/min，圆碟旋转速度为 5 000 r/min，使溶液在碟上铺展成均匀的液膜，液膜运行至碟缘被高速剪切成微滴，微滴飞旋进入气流场中，在液 - 气两相之间溶剂快速挥发，微滴逐渐固化成球。待微滴全部自然沉降至收集盘内后，收集并贮存于密闭干燥器内。

3. 质量评价

质量评价参照"五、（一）3."项的操作。

注意事项

（1）采用乳化-溶剂挥发法制备微球时，PVA 浓度决定了乳化能力，浓度较高时乳化能力较强，微球较易粘连；浓度较低时乳化能力较弱，微球粒径较大。

（2）采用乳化-溶剂挥发法制备微球时，适宜的搅拌速度能使微球粒径分布均匀。在低搅拌速度下，体系分散性差；而搅拌过快则易产生较多泡沫，产率降低。

（3）采用 UPPS 制备微球时，需要选择合适的供液速度。供液速度过慢，溶液不能连续供应至圆碟表面；供液速度过快，产物容易聚集粘连。

（4）采用 UPPS 制备微球时，需要选择合适的转速。转速较低时，产生的微滴粒径较大且不易干燥；转速较高时，液体在碟面上铺展得较快，导致产生丝状物。

六、实验结果与讨论

（一）石杉碱甲 PLGA 微球的制备（乳化-溶剂挥发法）

1. 外观形态
在显微镜下观察并描述微球的形态。

2. 粒径及其分布
记录所制备微球的平均粒径及其粒度分布，画出粒径分布直方图和粒径分布曲线。

3. 处方因素对微球质量的影响
（1）石杉碱甲标准曲线。以石杉碱甲浓度为横坐标，以峰面积为纵坐标，绘制石杉碱甲标准曲线。

（2）水相中乳化剂的含量对微球质量的影响（表 4 - 8）。

表 4 - 8　水相中乳化剂的含量对微球质量的影响

PVA/%	粒径/μm	跨距	载药量/%	包封率/%
1				
2				
3				

（3）油相中聚合物的浓度对微球质量的影响（表4-9）。

表4-9 油相中聚合物的浓度对微球质量的影响

PLGA 浓度/%	粒径/μm	跨距	载药量/%	包封率/%
5				
10				
20				

（二）超细微粒制备系统制备 PLGA 微球

分别测定微球粒径及其分布、载药量、包封率等指标，并与传统方法制备的微球进行比较。

七、思考题

（1）PLGA 作为微球骨架材料具有什么优势？

（2）本实验制备微球采用的 O/W 乳化-溶剂挥发法适用于什么类型的药物？

（3）结合实验结果，分析影响 O/W 乳化-溶剂挥发法制备微球质量的处方和工艺因素有哪些？

参考文献

［1］付寒，温新国，王周华，等. 超微粒制备系统制备利培酮长效注射微球［J］.中国新药杂志，2012，21（7）：795-799.

［2］WEN X G, PENG X S, HAN F, et al. Preparation and in vitro evaluation of silk fibroin microspheres produced by a novel ultra-fine particle processing system［J］. Int J Pharm, 2011（416）: 195-201.

［3］高萍. 石杉碱甲生物可降解长效注射微球的研究［D］.沈阳：沈阳药科大学，2006.

［4］国家药典委员会. 中华人民共和国药典［M］.北京：中国医药科技出版社，2020.

实验四　可溶性微针的制备及评价

一、实验目的

（1）掌握离心法制备可溶性微针。

（2）熟悉可溶性微针的评价方法。

二、实验原理

微针（microneedles）是一种新型的物理促渗制剂，由多个长 10～2 000 μm 的微型针头以阵列的方式连接在基座上构成，是一种结合皮下注射与经皮给药贴片双重优点的微创透皮给药系统。微针可在表皮形成微孔道，直接突破角质层的屏障，大大提高小分子及大分子药物的经皮渗透率。微针在刺入皮肤后不易触及皮肤深处的痛觉神经，只对皮肤造成轻度的物理损伤，实现无痛或微痛递药。

微针通常分为固体实心微针（solid microneedles）、涂层微针（coated microneedles）、空心微针（hollow microneedles）和可溶性微针（dissolving microneedles）等 4 种。可溶性微针一般由生物可降解的高分子材料制备而成，结构分为起支撑作用的基底层和装载药物的针尖层。可溶性微针的针尖层必须具有较好的机械性能以保证针体在刺入皮肤的过程中不会变形或断裂。因此，针尖层材料的选择至关重要。单一材料往往难以同时具有较好的硬度与韧性，为提高机械性能可以多种材料合用。

可溶性微针阵列刺入皮肤后，药物随着针尖的降解而逐渐释放。其制备简单，载药量高，且具有较好的生物相容性，无须担心针头在皮内折断而造成的安全隐患。目前，可溶性微针被广泛应用于药物、化妆品及诊断试剂等的经皮递送。

三、预习思考

（1）预习实验内容，熟悉离心法制备可溶性微针的流程。
（2）查阅资料，了解实验中所用的微针针尖材料的基本性质。
（3）查阅资料，了解物性分析仪的用途和用于机械强度的测定原理。

四、实验材料与仪器

1. 实验试剂与试药
聚二甲基硅氧烷（PDMS）及固化剂、右旋糖酐（DEX）、聚乙烯吡咯烷酮（PVP）K-30、透明质酸钠（HA）（分子量为 3～10 kDa）、生理盐水、台盼蓝、艾塞那肽、去离子水、三氟乙酸、乙腈。

2. 实验仪器
天平、离心机、真空干燥箱、烘箱、电推剪、电动剃须刀、眼科镊、眼科弯剪、物性分析仪、0.22 μm 微孔滤膜、高效液相色谱仪、干燥器、放大镜、显微镜。

3. 实验动物
SD 大鼠。

五、实验内容

（一）空白可溶性微针的制备

1. 微针阳模的制备

设计微针阳模的模具尺寸、针数、针型和针间距，并通过专业软件 CAD 绘制模具平面图和立体图。对照 CAD 设计图进行数控编程，根据程序编码，运算并转换成指令后，控制精密数控机床系统，一般以金属为模具材料，通过粗、中、精多步骤重复性加工，完成微针阳模的制造（图 4 - 1）。

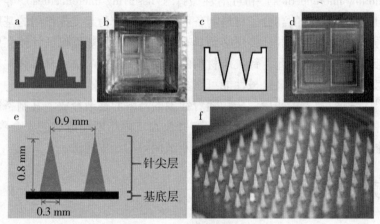

图 4 - 1 可溶性微针阳模

阳膜结构示意图（a）和实物图（b）；阴模的结构示意图（c）和实物图（d）；
可溶性微针贴片的结构示意图（e）和成品图（f）。

2. 微针阴模的制备

取 PDMS 与固化剂以 10∶1 的比例混合并搅拌均匀。然后，将一定量的 PDMS 混合液倒入微针阳模，并将模具置于真空干燥箱中真空脱气 20 min，以除去气泡。随后把微针阳模置于 80 ℃烘箱中加热 2 h。待 PDMS 完全固化后，取出阳模，小心分离即得阴模。

3. 微针针体材料溶液的配制

选择不同的高分子材料（DEX、PVP 和 HA）作为微针针体材料，称取 1 g 高分子材料，加入 4 mL 去离子水，常温搅拌至完全溶解，制得微针针体材料溶液。

4. 可溶性微针的制备

取 0.30 mL 微针针体材料溶液于阴模中，然后将阴模置于离心机的摇篮中，以4 000 r/min 的转速在 4 ℃离心 5 min，使针体溶液填满阴模的微孔道。把离心好的模具置于干燥器中常温干燥 72 h，待完全干燥后，用镊子轻轻取出微针，适当修剪针尖基底层边缘，置于干燥器中保存，待用。

5. 质量评价

（1）外观形态。

采用放大镜和显微镜观察所制备的微针贴片。

（2）机械强度测定。

采用物性分析仪考察可溶性微针在外力作用下的针尖受力情况，以确定其机械强度。将微针针尖朝上，平放于物性分析仪的载物台上，设定探头以 0.01 mm/s 的速度缓慢下降，当探头接触到针尖并检测到触发力（设定为 5.0 g）后，探头的下降速率调整为 0.05 mm/s。随着探头缓慢下降，压力逐渐上升，针尖被进一步压缩，直至断裂，探头随即以 0.5 mm/s 的速度上升并离开针尖。软件记录此过程的压力变化，以位移为横坐标，探头所受的压力为纵坐标，绘制压力 – 位移曲线。

（3）微针穿刺性能研究。

大鼠离体皮肤制备：取 200～250 g SD 大鼠，颈椎脱臼处死，用电推剪去除背部长毛，电动剃须刀刮剃短毛，然后剥离背部皮肤。把皮肤角质层向下固定在平板上，眼科镊和眼科弯剪配合使用，仔细剥除脂肪层和结缔组织。用生理盐水清洗皮肤后，铺平，用锡纸包裹，置于 –20 ℃冷冻保存，备用。

将冷冻保存的鼠皮于生理盐水中解冻后拭干，角质层向上平铺于 PDMS 材质的平面上，以模拟皮肤实际的弹性和硬度。取出微针，用大拇指以一定力度将其按压于皮肤上，停留 30 s 后，用医用胶布固定，10 min 后拔出微针，用 0.4% 台盼蓝溶液浸染皮肤表面，10 min 后除去皮肤表面的染色剂，并用棉球蘸生理盐水擦拭干净，观察皮肤表面染色小孔的情况，拍摄照片。

（4）针尖溶解性研究。

取不同高分子材料制得的微针若干，分别按压于新鲜的离体去毛大鼠皮肤上，每片微针按压 30 s 后开始计时，分别于 0 min、10 min 和 30 min 后取出，用显微镜观察可溶性微针的针尖溶解情况。每个时间点重复 3 次，根据针尖剩余的高度，绘制可溶性微针针尖在皮肤内的溶解时间曲线。

（二）艾塞那肽可溶性微针的制备

1. 含药针尖溶液的配制

按处方称取艾塞那肽，用去离子水溶解后，加入 DEX，充分搅拌使其完全溶解，制得含药针尖溶液。

改变针尖溶液中药物和高分子材料的量，通过测定微针贴片的机械强度评价制备好的不同微针。不同微针的针尖处方如表 4 – 10 所示。

表 4 – 10　含药针尖溶液的制备处方

处方编号	艾塞那肽/g	DEX/g	去离子水/mL
F1	0.2	1	4
F2	0.4	1	4
F3	0.2	2	4
F4	0.4	2	4

2. 基底溶液的配制

将 5.0 g DEX 加入 10 mL 去离子水中，搅拌均匀并溶胀过夜，再充分搅匀，以 2 000 r/min 的转速离心 1 min，除去气泡，制得基底层溶液。

3. 可溶性微针的制备

取 0.2 mL 针尖溶液于阴模中，然后将阴模置于离心机的摇篮中，以 4 000 r/min 的转速在 4 ℃离心 10 min，使针尖溶液填满阴模的微孔道。取出阴模，使用刮铲充分刮走残留在阴模表面过量的针尖溶液后，加入适量微针基底溶液，于离心机中以 2 000 r/min 的转速在 4 ℃离心 3 min，使基底溶液均匀覆盖微孔道。把离心好的模具置于干燥器中常温干燥 72 h，待完全干燥后，用镊子轻轻取出微针，适当修剪针尖基底层边缘，置于干燥器中保存，待用。

4. 质量评价

（1）外观形态、机械强度、微针穿刺性能与针尖溶解性研究。方法同上文"五、（一）5."项的质量评价部分。

（2）微针含药量测定。标准曲线的绘制：精密称取艾塞那肽 7.5 mg 于 5 mL 容量瓶中，用流动相 A 溶解并稀释成浓度为 1.5 mg/mL 的艾塞那肽贮备液。精密量取不同体积的艾塞那肽贮备液，分别稀释成终浓度为 0.03 mg/mL、0.06 mg/mL、0.12 mg/mL、0.18 mg/mL、0.30 mg/mL、0.60 mg/mL、1.20 mg/mL 的艾塞那肽标准工作液。依次取上述各浓度标准工作液，过 0.22 μm 微孔滤膜后，按照色谱条件进样，进行色谱分析，记录峰面积。以峰面积对艾塞那肽浓度进行线性回归，绘制标准曲线。

高效液相色谱条件：色谱柱为 Gemini-NX（C18 110A，250 mm × 4.60 mm，5 μm，Phenomenex 公司）；流动相 A 为含 0.1% 三氟乙酸的水溶液，流动相 B 为含 0.1% 三氟乙酸的乙腈溶液；流速为 1.0 mL/min；柱温为 30 ℃；进样量为 20 μL；检测波长为 220 nm。采用梯度洗脱法进行检测，流动相的梯度洗脱程序遵循表 4-11。

表 4-11 流动相梯度洗脱程序

时间/min	流动相 A/%	流动相 B/%
0.00	70	30
20.00	50	50
20.01	0	100
30.00	70	30
35.00	70	30

微针含药量测定：取艾塞那肽可溶性微针，剪成小块后，置于离心管中，用 2 mL 去离子水溶解，并加入 12 mL 流动相 A 进行稀释，用 0.22 μm 微孔滤膜过滤后按照预定的色谱条件进行进样测定，记录峰面积，根据标准曲线计算溶液中艾塞那肽的浓度，并由此计算微针中艾塞那肽的总含量。

六、实验结果与讨论

1. 可溶性微针针尖辅料的选择

通过考察不同高分子材料制备所得的空白可溶性微针的外观形态、机械强度、微针穿刺性能和针尖溶解性，评价哪一种辅料更适合用作针尖基质材料。

2. 微针中药物的含量测定

为了优选出最佳处方，测定采用不同处方制备得到的艾塞那肽可溶性微针的针尖含药量，并将结果填入表4-12。

表4-12　载药微针针尖含药量

处方编号	微针含药量/μg
F1	
F2	
F3	
F4	

七、思考题

（1）可溶性微针相比于传统经皮给药剂型有哪些优势？

（2）简述微针的分类及各类微针的优缺点。

（3）影响可溶性微针针尖载药量的因素有哪些？

（4）结合PDMS的性质，简述选择其作为微针阴模材料的原因。

（5）理想的针尖基质材料需要满足什么特点，若选用单一的针尖材料无法获得综合性能较好的微针针尖，可采取哪些改进策略？

参考文献

[1] WANG Q Q, YAO G T, DONG P, et al. Investigation on fabrication process of dissolving microneedle arrays to improve effective needle drug distribution [J]. Eur J Pharm Biophar, 2015, 66: 148-156.

[2] LIN S Q, CAI B Z, QUAN G L, et al. Novel strategy for immunomodulation: Dissolving microneedle array encapsulating thymopentin fabricated by modified two-step molding technology [J]. Eur J Pharm Biophar, 2018, 122: 104-112.

吸入粉雾剂的制备及评价

一、实验目的

（1）掌握喷雾干燥法和气流粉碎法的基本操作。
（2）熟悉吸入粉雾剂的质量评价方法。
（3）了解吸入粉雾剂的制备方法。

二、实验原理

1. 吸入制剂

吸入制剂，系指一种或几种活性药物，溶解或分散于合适的介质中，以蒸汽或气溶胶形式递送至肺部发挥局部或全身作用的液体（吸入气雾剂和雾化吸入溶液）或固体制剂（吸入粉雾剂）。该类制剂往往需要特定的装置将药物通过粉状或雾状等形式经口腔传送至呼吸道或肺部。

2. 吸入粉雾剂

吸入粉雾剂（dry powder inhalation，DPI），系指固体微粉化药物单独或与合适载体混合后，以胶囊、泡囊或多剂量贮库形式，采用特制的吸入装置，由患者吸入雾化药物至肺部的制剂。与吸入气雾剂和雾化吸入溶液相比，吸入粉雾剂具有以下特点：①患者主动吸入药粉，顺应性好，不存在给药时配合的困难；②无抛射剂，可避免对环境污染和对呼吸道刺激；③药物按胶囊预先分装，剂量准确，无超剂量风险；④不含有机溶媒，对黏膜和呼吸道无刺激等。

吸入粉雾剂的吸入效果很大程度上受粉体粒子的粒径、外观形态等性质的影响。吸入粉雾剂粒子常为形态不规则颗粒，因此我们可采用空气动力学直径（aerodynamic diameter，d_a）来表征吸入粉雾剂的粒子大小，根据式（4-5-1）计算：

$$d_a = d_e \left(\frac{\rho_p}{\rho_o} \cdot X \right)^{\frac{1}{2}} \tag{4-5-1}$$

式中，d_e为球形等效粒径；ρ_p为颗粒聚集密度，$\rho_o = 1 \text{ g/cm}^3$；$X$为动态形态因子，粒子为球形时，$X=1$。通常认为，当颗粒的空气动力学直径为 $1 \sim 5$ μm 时，易吸入肺部，当 d_a 小于 2 μm 时，易进入肺泡。

根据 2020 版《中国药典》规定，应对吸入粉雾剂含量均匀度、递送剂量均一性、微细粒子剂量（fine particle dose，以 FPD 表示）及其在递送剂量中的比例（fine particle fraction，以 *FPF* 表示）、微生物限度等进行考察，对于多剂量吸入粉雾剂，还需对其总吸次进行考察。

3. 吸入粉雾剂的制备方法

由于吸入粉雾剂的吸入效果与粒径大小有密切关系，药物的微粉化处理是制备吸入粉雾剂的一个关键步骤。目前常用的微粉化工艺有气流粉碎法、喷雾干燥法、研磨法、超临界制备法和结晶法等。

喷雾干燥法（spray drying）可将液体原料直接转变成干燥粒子，易于实现大工业生产，是近年来应用最广泛的微粉化技术。该法技术灵活，可通过控制工艺参数，如更换喷嘴或调节气流量等，制备得到不同粒径和不同形态的粒子。

气流粉碎法（jet milling）是常用的物料微粉化处理方法。该法处理后的物料颗粒粒径较小且分布均一，且由于高压空气从喷嘴喷出时产生焦耳－汤姆逊冷却效应，该法也适用于热敏物料和低熔点物料的粉碎。

经微粉化处理的颗粒往往具有较高的表面能，容易发生聚集。为改善吸入粉雾剂的流动性和分散性，获得更高的剂量准确性和更好的吸入效果，往往需要加入载体颗粒。

三、预习思考

（1）查阅相关资料，了解其他的微粉化处理方法。
（2）相较其他制剂，吸入制剂有哪些特点？
（3）查阅相关资料，简述异丙托溴铵和布地奈德的理化性质。

四、实验材料与仪器

1. 实验试剂与试药
异丙托溴铵、布地奈德、乳糖载体 Inhalac@251、蒸馏水、无水乙醇。
2. 实验仪器
天平、激光粒度分析仪、新一代粒子撞击器、高效液相色谱仪、喷雾干燥机、微型气流粉碎机、烧杯、量筒、容量瓶、3#胶囊壳。

五、实验内容

（一）胶囊型异丙托溴铵吸入粉雾剂的制备及评价[①]

1. 异丙托溴铵药物微粉化处理
将约 2 g 异丙托溴铵溶解于 200 mL 蒸馏水中，接入 SD-1000 喷雾干燥机进样器。喷

---

① 由于批量过小，本节对胶囊型粉雾剂进行的混合和填装操作均为实验室条件下的操作，与实际工业生产操作不同。

雾干燥的参数设置如下：喷嘴直径 0.71 mm，雾化压力 50 kPa，进风温度 140 ℃，气流量 0.60 m³/h，在此条件下调整泵液速度，使对应的出风温度稳定为 80 ℃。喷干结束后收集样品瓶中的样品即得微粉化的异丙托溴铵，干燥保存。

2. 胶囊型异丙托溴铵吸入粉雾剂的制备

以喷雾干燥方法处理得到的药物微粉，制备两种胶囊型异丙托溴铵吸入粉雾剂。异丙托溴铵吸入粉雾剂 1：直接将药物微粉装入 3# 明胶胶囊中；异丙托溴铵吸入粉雾剂 2：取 1 g 微粉化药物，与 10 g 乳糖载体 Inhalac@ 251 均匀混合后装入 3# 明胶胶囊中。精密称量，使每颗胶囊内容物为（10.0 ± 0.5）mg，填装 30 颗胶囊，于干燥环境保存，备用。

3. 粒径分布

采用动态光散射法（干法）测定异丙托溴铵吸入粉雾剂 1 和 2 的粒径。本样品测定时，Malvern 2000 激光粒度分析仪参数设置如下：分散压力 3.5 bar，遮光度 0.5% ～ 5%。每个样品平行测定 3 次。

4. 递送剂量均一性测试

参照《中国药典》2020 版通则 0111 吸入制剂中的"吸入粉雾剂"项下"递送剂量均一性"方法进行测试，测定方法和测定装置详情见附录ⅢC。

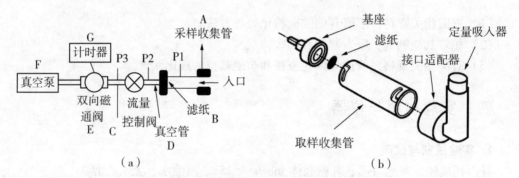

图 4 - 2 递送剂量均一性测试装置与组装结构

a：递送剂量均一性测试装置；b：装置组装结构。

1）安装测试装置（图 4 - 2）。装置入口端安装合适的适配器，确保吸入剂吸嘴端口与样品收集端口平齐。在基座内放入圆形滤纸，固定于取样收集管的一端。收集管基座端口与真空泵相连，另一端通过适配器连接吸入装置。

2）开启真空泵，打开双向磁通阀，调节流量控制阀，使吸入装置前后的压力差（P_1）为 4.0 kPa。取下吸入装置，在装置入口连接流量计，测定离开流量计的体积流量 Q_{out}。对于测定进入体积流量 Q_{in} 的流量计，可按式（4 - 5 - 2）换算：

$$Q_{out} = \frac{Q_{in} \times P_0}{P_0 - \Delta P} \quad\quad (4 - 5 - 2)$$

式中，P_0 为大气压，ΔP 为流量计前后压差。

若测得 Q_{out} 大于 100 L/min，调节流量至 100 L/min；若流速小于 100 L/min，保持流速不变，流速记为 Q_{out}。按式（4 - 5 - 3）计算抽气时间 t：

$$t = \frac{4 \times 60}{Q_{\text{out}}} \qquad (4-5-3)$$

记录 P_2 及 P_3 值，P_3/P_2 应不大于 0.5。

3）将待测胶囊 1 颗装入吸入装置，按压装置刺破胶囊。再次按图 4-2 安装测试装置。开启真空泵，抽气。关闭真空泵，取下吸入装置。以蒸馏水清洗滤纸和收集管内部，合并清洗液后定容至 50 mL，测定各溶液中的含药量。重复上述过程，每种胶囊测试 10 颗。

4）结果判定。符合下列条件之一者，可判定为符合规定：

（1）10 个测定结果中，至少 9 个测定值在平均值的 75%～125%，且全部在平均值的 65～135%。

（2）10 个测定结果中，若有 2～3 个测定值超出平均值的 75%～125%，则另取 20 颗胶囊测定。30 个测定结果中，超出 75%～125% 的测定值不多于 3 个，且全部都在平均值的 65%～135%。

5. 沉积分布测试

参照《中国药典》2020 版通则 0951 吸入制剂微细粒子空气动力学特性测试法进行沉积分布测试。测定方法和测定装置详见附录 ⅢC。

安装测试装置：在预分离器中央的收集杯内加入 15 mL 蒸馏水，扣紧预分离器，接着将撞击器主体、预分离器和直角模拟喉依次连接，使之成为密封系统。保持吸入器与直角模拟喉在同一水平轴线。在模拟喉入口处接流量计，设置气流量 Q_{out} 和抽气时间 t 与"五、（一）4. 2）"项的一致。

取下流量计，接上适配器和吸入装置。取待测胶囊 1 颗，放入给药装置中，按压装置刺破胶囊，开启真空泵，抽气 1 次，取下给药装置，取出待测胶囊。重复以上操作，每种胶囊测试 10 颗，关闭电源，拆除装置。以蒸馏水为收集液，分别收集吸入装置和适配器、预分离器、直角模拟喉、第 1 阶段至第 7 阶段及微孔收集器（MOC）中的粉末，测定各部分药物含量。根据不同气流量，计算有效截止粒径小于 5 μm 的收集盘（表 4-13）中药物总量及其比例，绘制沉积分布图。测试重复 3 次。

表 4-13　不同 Q_{out} 下各盘的有效截止粒径

$Q_{\text{out}}/(\text{L} \cdot \text{min}^{-1})$	有效截止粒径/μm							
	第 1 阶段	第 2 阶段	第 3 阶段	第 4 阶段	第 5 阶段	第 6 阶段	第 7 阶段	MOC
60	8.06	4.46	2.82	1.66	0.94	0.55	0.34	0
15	14.10	8.61	5.39	3.30	2.08	1.36	0.98	0

6. 异丙托溴铵标准曲线的建立

精密称取异丙托溴铵 25.0 mg，用蒸馏水溶解并定容至 50 mL 作为贮备液。精密量取贮备液适量，分别用蒸馏水稀释至浓度为 5.0 μg/mL、20.0 μg/mL、40.0 μg/mL、60.0 μg/mL 和 80.0 μg/mL 的溶液，采用高效液相色谱法，各进样 20 μL，记录峰面积。以药物浓度对峰面积进行线性回归，得异丙托溴铵标准曲线。异丙托溴铵高效液相色谱条件如下：以十八烷基硅烷键合硅胶为填充剂；以磷酸盐缓冲液（用磷酸、0.4% 三乙胺调节 pH 至 3.0）– 乙腈（84∶16）为流动相；检测波长为 205 nm；流速为 1.0 mL/min；进样量为 20 μL。

（二）胶囊型布地奈德吸入粉雾剂的制备及表征

1. 布地奈德药物微粉化处理

取约 5 g 布地奈德，在干燥环境下缓慢加入 AO 型气流粉碎机进料斗进行粉碎。气流粉碎的工艺参数设置如下：研磨压力 4.0 kPa，饲粉压力 5.0 kPa。粉碎完成后收集，于干燥环境下保存。

2. 胶囊型布地奈德吸入粉雾剂的制备

以气流粉碎方法处理得到的药物微粉，制备 2 种胶囊型布地奈德吸入粉雾剂。

（1）布地奈德吸入粉雾剂 1。直接将制得的微粉化药物装入 3# 明胶胶囊中。

（2）布地奈德吸入粉雾剂 2。取 1 g 微粉化药物，与 10 g 乳糖载体 Inhalac@251 均匀混合后装入 3# 明胶胶囊中。精密称量使每颗胶囊内容物为（10.0 ± 0.5）mg，填装 30 颗胶囊，于干燥环境保存，备用。

3. 粒径分布、递送剂量均一性和沉积分布测试

胶囊评价参照"五、（一）"中的操作，仅将所需溶剂由蒸馏水变更为无水乙醇。

4. 布地奈德标准曲线的建立

精密称取布地奈德 25.0 mg，用蒸馏水溶解并定容至 50 mL 作为贮备液，用无水乙醇溶解并定容，得贮备液。精密量取贮备液适量，分别用无水乙醇稀释至浓度为 5.0 μg/mL、20.0 μg/mL、40.0 μg/mL、60.0 μg/mL、80.0 μg/mL 和 100.0 μg/mL 的溶液，采用高效液相色谱法，各进样 20 μL，记录峰面积。以药物浓度对峰面积进行线性回归，得布地奈德标准曲线。布地奈德高效液相色谱条件如下：以十八烷基硅烷键合硅胶为填充剂；以水 – 乙腈（30∶70）为流动相；检测波长为 240 nm；流速为 1.0 mL/min；进样量为 20 μL。

> **注意事项**

喷雾干燥结束后，先降低进风温度，使仪器温度降至 40 ℃ 以下再关闭仪器，以免设备散热不良而损坏。

六、实验结果与讨论

（一）胶囊型异丙托溴铵吸入粉雾剂的制备

1. 外观性状

描述制备的吸入粉雾剂的外观性状。

2. 粒径分布

记录所制备吸入粉雾剂的平均粒径及其粒度分布。

3. 递送剂量均一性

记录吸入粉雾剂的药物递送量并计算平均值。

4. 沉积分布

（1）异丙托溴铵标准曲线的绘制。以异丙托溴铵浓度为横坐标，以峰面积为纵坐标，绘制异丙托溴铵标准曲线。

（2）绘制沉积分布图，计算 FPD 和 FPF。记录吸入粉雾剂在各级的药物沉积量，绘制沉积分布图并计算 FPD 和 FPF（表4-14）。

表4-14　异丙托溴铵吸入粉雾剂粒径、FPD 和 FPF

组别	$d_{0.1}/\mu m$	$d_{0.5}/\mu m$	$d_{0.9}/\mu m$	FPD/mg	$FPF/\%$
异丙托溴铵吸入粉雾剂1					
异丙托溴铵吸入粉雾剂2					

（二）胶囊型布地奈德吸入粉雾剂的制备

1. 外观性状

描述制备的吸入粉雾剂内容物的外观形态特征。

2. 粒径分布

记录所制备吸入粉雾剂的平均粒径及其粒度分布。

3. 递送剂量均一性

记录吸入粉雾剂的药物递送量并计算平均值。

4. 沉积分布

（1）布地奈德标准曲线。以布地奈德浓度为横坐标，以峰面积为纵坐标，绘制布地奈德标准曲线。

（2）绘制沉积分布图，计算 FPD 和 FPF。计算吸入粉雾剂在各级的药物沉积量，绘制沉积分布图，并计算 FPD 和 FPF（表4-15）。

表4-15　布地奈德吸入粉雾剂粒径、FPD 和 FPF

组别	$d_{0.1}/\mu m$	$d_{0.5}/\mu m$	$d_{0.9}/\mu m$	FPD/mg	$FPF/\%$
布地奈德吸入粉雾剂1					
布地奈德吸入粉雾剂2					

七、思考题

（1）吸入粉雾剂、吸入气雾剂和雾化吸入溶液有什么差异？它们的质量评价有哪些不同？

（2）吸入制剂在选用辅料时应注意哪些方面的问题？

（3）除本文介绍的两种方法外，还有哪些对药物进行微粉化处理的方法？请简述其中一种。

参考文献

［1］国家药典委员会. 中华人民共和国药典：四部［M］.北京：中国医药科技出版社，2020.

［2］周建平，唐星. 工业药剂学［M］.北京：人民卫生出版社，2014：257－271.

［3］PENG T T, ZHANG X J, HUANG Y, et al. Nanoporous mannitol carrier prepared by non-organic solvent spray drying technique to enhance the aerosolization performance for dry powder inhalation［J］. Scientific Report, 2017（7）：46517.

［4］刘骥飞，戴剑锋，贾钰泽，等. 气流破碎在高纯碳酸锂粉末粒径优化中的应用［J］.化工进展，2018（11）：4162－4167.

实验六　骨架缓释片的制备及评价

一、实验目的

（1）掌握常用骨架缓释片的类型与缓释原理。

（2）熟悉常用骨架缓释片的材料。

（3）熟悉常用骨架缓释片的制备方法。

（4）了解骨架缓释片的质量评价方法。

二、实验原理

骨架型缓释片（matrix tablets）是指药物和一种或多种惰性固体骨架材料通过压制或融合技术制成片状的制剂。一般缓释骨架的类型可分为亲水凝胶型骨架、不溶性骨架和生物溶蚀性骨架。其中，亲水凝胶型骨架片是以亲水性聚合物或天然胶类为骨架材料制成的水凝胶型缓释片。

亲水凝胶型骨架材料，遇水能膨胀形成凝胶阻滞层，控制药物的释放速率。常见的亲水凝胶骨架材料包括羟丙甲基纤维素（HPMC）、海藻酸钠（SA）、壳聚糖（CS）和聚乙烯醇（PVA）等。同一种骨架材料，根据其官能团的取代度、平均分子量和分子量分布等的不同，可以分为不同型号。其黏度和水化速率也具有显著性差异。

一般认为，亲水凝胶型骨架片中药物释放是药物扩散与骨架溶蚀相结合的过程。药物释放主要受骨架材料种类、用量及比例影响。释放介质首先润湿片剂表面，形成凝胶层，使表面药物溶出。然后，骨架材料吸水膨胀形成具有黏性的凝胶层，阻滞药物在凝胶层的扩散。随着凝胶层的不断水化，片剂外层骨架逐渐溶蚀，内部形成凝胶，直至水分向片芯渗透致骨架完全溶蚀，药物释放完全。一般情况下，骨架型缓释片所装载药物的溶解性不同，其释药机制也不同。对于水溶性药物，其释药主要以扩散和骨架溶蚀为主；而对于难溶性药物，释药主要以骨架溶蚀为主。

亲水凝胶型骨架片的制备工艺一般分为湿法制粒压片和粉末直接压片。湿法制粒压片通过制粒可改善物料的流动性及可压性，提高物料混合的均匀性，防止物料分层，减少片重差异，提高含量均匀度，但能源消耗较多，劳力消耗大，时间消耗久，生产效率较低。粉末直接压片制备工艺简单，有利于片剂生产的连续化与自动化，适用于湿热不稳定的药物，但本法对物料要求较高，压片的粉末需有适宜的粒度、结晶状态、可压性、黏结性及流动性。

三、预习思考

(1) 列举 5 个市售的骨架缓释片品种，说明它们的类型。
(2) 查阅相关资料，简述拉莫三嗪的理化性质。
(3) 简这片剂质量评价相关知识。
(4) 简述常用的缓释骨架辅料及特点。

四、实验材料与仪器

1. 实验试剂与试药
拉莫三嗪、羟丙基甲基纤维素（HPMC K4M CR、K100 LV CR）、直压乳糖、微粉硅胶、硬脂酸镁、甲醇、醋酸铵、冰醋酸。

2. 实验仪器
80 目筛、旋转式压片机、天平、超声波清洗仪、溶出仪、0.45 μm 微孔滤膜、高效液相色谱仪。

五、实验内容

（一）拉莫三嗪骨架缓释片的制备

1. 处方

拉莫三嗪	5 g
HPMC K4M CR	7.5 g
HPMC K100 LV CR	2.5 g
直压乳糖	15 g

微粉硅胶	0.3 g
硬脂酸镁	0.3 g
共制成	100 片

2. 实验步骤

将拉莫三嗪与辅料分别过 80 目筛，按处方量称取拉莫三嗪、HPMC K4M CR、HPMC K100 LV CR 和直压乳糖，混合均匀，加入微粉硅胶与硬脂酸镁混匀后，粉末直接压片。

（二）拉莫三嗪骨架缓释片释放度的测定

1. 标准曲线的绘制

精密称取干燥的拉莫三嗪对照品约 25 mg 于 25 mL 容量瓶中，加甲醇适量振摇分散，超声 15 min，放冷，定容。精密量取贮备液适量，分别用甲醇稀释至浓度为 5.0 $\mu g/mL$、10.0 $\mu g/mL$、15.0 $\mu g/mL$、20.0 $\mu g/mL$ 和 25.0 $\mu g/mL$ 的对照品溶液，摇匀。采用 HPLC 法于 210 nm 测定不同浓度对照品溶液的峰面积，以峰面积对浓度绘制标准曲线。

2. 拉莫三嗪骨架缓释片释放曲线的绘制

取拉莫三嗪骨架缓释片，采用 0.2 mol/L pH 为 6.8 的磷酸缓冲液（含 0.5% SDS）900 mL 为溶出介质，温度（37.0±0.5 ℃），桨法，转速 50 r/min。分别于第 1 h、2 h、3 h、4 h、6 h、8 h、10 h 和 12 h 各取溶出杯中溶液 5 mL，经 0.45 μm 微孔滤膜过滤，取续滤液，采用 HPLC 法测定拉莫三嗪的含量，计算体外累积百分释放度，绘制释放曲线。注意及时补充相同体积和温度的磷酸缓冲液至溶出介质中。

高效液相色谱条件：色谱柱为 Gemini C18 反相色谱柱（4.6 mm×250 mm）；流动相为甲醇–醋酸铵缓冲盐（冰醋酸调节 pH=4.5）（40∶60）；检测波长 210 nm；柱温为 40 ℃；流速 1.0 mL/min；进样量 20 μL。

（三）处方组成对拉莫三嗪骨架缓释片释放度的影响

HPMC 比例对释放度的影响：保持处方中 HPMC K4M CR 和 HPMC K100 LV CR 总量不变，考察二者质量比分别为 1∶1、3∶1 和 5∶1 对缓释片释放度的影响。

填充剂用量对释放度的影响：保持处方中其他组分及比例不变，考察直压乳糖用量分别为 9 g、15 g 和 21 g 对缓释片释放度的影响。

注意事项

本实验通过考察不同组分用量对拉莫三嗪骨架缓释片释放的影响，旨在让学生了解辅料对骨架缓释片药物释放的影响。如果涉及仿制药处方筛选，往往采用计算相似因子（f_2）的方法，来评价参比制剂与受试制剂的相似性，相关内容参考附录ⅢD，将结果填入表 4-16 中。

表 4 – 16　各模型的拟合结果

模型	拟合方程	R^2
零级释放		
一级释放		
Higuchi 方程		

六、实验结果与讨论

拉莫三嗪骨架缓释片制备及评价

1. 外观形态
观察并记录片剂完整度、光泽、色泽均匀度等。

2. 释放度
（1）对"五、（二）"中所得释放数据进行曲线拟合，拟合方程参考附录ⅢD。

（2）测定不同辅料及用量制得的拉莫三嗪骨架缓释片的释放曲线，对结果进行分析讨论。

七、思考题

（1）请分析本实验处方中不同组成的作用。

（2）试分析拉莫三嗪骨架缓释片可能的释放机制。

参考文献

［1］MA C，HUANG Z W，ZHU Y M，et al. Production and in vitro evaluation of a lamotrigine extended release tablet based on a controlled-porosity osmotic pump system.［J］. Pharmazie，2017，72（9）：511 – 517.

［2］国家药典委员会. 中华人民共和国药典：四部［M］.北京：中国医药科技出版社，2020.

实验七 微乳的制备及评价

一、实验目的

(1) 熟悉伪三元相图的绘制方法及微乳区域的确定。
(2) 熟悉微乳的制备方法。
(3) 了解微乳的质量检查方法。

二、实验原理

微乳（microemulsion）是由油、水、乳化剂及助乳化剂组成的各向同性的热力学稳定体系。按结构，微乳可分为水包油型（O/W），油包水型（W/O）和双连续相型。微乳液滴大小通常在 $10 \sim 100$ nm 之间，外观呈透明或半透明，可在较大温度范围内保持热力学稳定，经热压灭菌或离心不分层。微乳在一定条件下可自发形成，无须外力做功。处方中大量的乳化剂和助乳化剂可在油水界面形成超低界面张力，有利于曲率半径很小的液滴形成。由于液滴内部同时存在亲油、亲水区域，微乳能增加难溶性药物的溶解度。

微乳的制备处方可通过伪三元相图得到。绘制含有乳化剂、助乳化剂、油和水四组分的伪三元相图时，通常将乳化剂/助乳化剂置于正三角形的一个顶点上，将油和水置于三角形的另外两个顶点。不同乳化剂和助乳化剂比例（K_m 值）对微乳形成的影响可通过绘制不同的相图进行研究。如图 4-3 所示，顶点上标"表面活性剂"，代表该点表面活性剂的含量是 100%。该顶点对面的直线则代表表面活性剂的含量是 0%。作其平行线将其与表面活性剂的距离分成 10 等份，从下到上各平行线分别代表含表面活性剂 10%、20%、30%……例如，图 4-3 中的点 P 含表面活性剂 50%、油 20%、水 30%。

微乳区域通常采用水滴定法绘制伪三元相图来确定：将乳化剂（包括助乳化剂）和油预先混匀，然后用水滴定。如图 4-4，A 和 B 代表表面活性剂和油的比例分别为 $1:4$ 和 $1:1$，用水滴定时表面活性剂和油的比例不变，滴定曲线从点 A 和点 B 指向水的顶点。假设分别滴定至点 M 和点 N 液体从澄清变浑浊，则点 M 和点 N 为相变点。继续改变表面活性剂和油比例（如 $1:9$，$1:6$……）进行滴定，可以得到多个相变点，连接各相变点，单相区即为微乳区。伪三相图可采用 Origin 软件进行绘制。

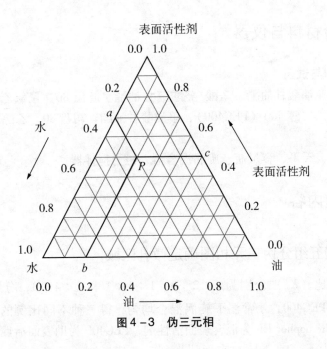

图 4 – 3 伪三元相

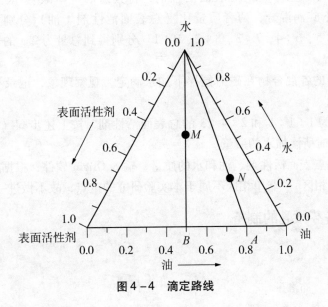

图 4 – 4 滴定路线

三、预习思考

（1）简述布洛芬的理化性质。
（2）简述滴定法绘制伪三元相图的流程。

四、实验材料与仪器

1. 实验试剂与试药

布洛芬、单亚油酸甘油酯、辛酸/癸酸三甘油酯、吐温 80、聚氧乙烯蓖麻油（Cremophor EL）、聚乙二醇 400（PEG400）、单油酸甘油酯、司盘 80、乙醇。

2. 实验仪器

烧杯、量筒、天平、容量瓶、旋涡混合器、磁力搅拌器。

五、实验内容

（一）绘制五组分伪三元相图确定微乳区域

（1）按质量比（K_m）分别为 4：2：3、1：1：1 和 2：4：3，分别称取吐温 80，Cremophor EL 和 PEG400，于常温下旋涡混合均匀，得三种不同比例的总表面活性剂。其中吐温 80 与 Cremophor EL 为混合表面活性剂，PEG400 为助表面活性剂。

（2）取 K_m 为 4：2：3 的总表面活性剂，将其与油（辛酸/癸酸三甘油酯，简称 GTCC）于常温下旋涡混合，两者质量比（总表面活性剂：油）分别为 1：9、2：8、3：7、4：6、5：5、6：4、7：3、8：2、9：1。分别得到总量为 2 g 的表面活性剂 – 油的混合物。

（3）将制得的各混合物在磁力搅拌下加水滴定，观察现象，记录相变点时滴加水的质量。

（4）取 K_m 为 1：1：1 和 2：4：3 的总表面活性剂，按上述步骤（2）和步骤（3）分别记录相变点时所滴加水的质量。

（5）将相变点表面活性剂、油和水的质量，输入 Origin 软件，根据相变点及连线确定微乳区域（单相区）。非单相区不属于本实验研究的重点，故不做进一步的划分。

（二）布洛芬微乳的制备

1. 处方

布洛芬	0.1 g
单亚油酸甘油酯（油）	0.3 g
辛酸/癸酸三甘油酯（油）	0.3 g
吐温 80（表面活性剂）	0.6 g
Cremophor EL（表面活性剂）	0.6 g
PEG400（表面活性剂）	1.2 g
蒸馏水	6.9 g

2. 实验步骤

单亚油酸甘油酯于 55 ℃加热熔融，加入辛酸/癸酸三甘油酯搅拌均匀。将布洛芬和混合表面活性剂加入油相中混合。在磁力搅拌下，将蒸馏水缓慢滴加入油相混合物中，形成微乳。

3. 质量检查

（1）外观性状。布洛芬微乳应呈透明或半透明略带乳光的无色液体。

（2）粒径。取微乳 100 μL，加 2 mL 水稀释，于激光粒度仪中测定粒径。

（3）离心稳定性。取微乳 1 mL 于 2 mL 离心管中，10 000 r/min 转速离心 15 min，观察微乳是否分层。

六、实验结果与讨论

（一）伪三元相图的绘制

1. $K_m = 4 : 2 : 3$

各成分滴加质量见表 4 – 17。

表 4 – 17　$K_m = 4 : 2 : 3$ 时各成分滴加质量

编号	混合表面活性剂/g	GTCC/g	水/g
1			
2			
3			
4			
5			
6			
7			
8			
9			

2. $K_m = 1 : 1 : 1$

各成分滴加质量见表 4 – 18。

表 4 – 18　$K_m = 1 : 1 : 1$ 时各成分滴加质量

编号	混合表面活性剂/g	GTCC/g	水/g
1			
2			
3			
4			
5			

续表 4 – 18

编号	混合表面活性剂/g	GTCC/g	水/g
6			
7			
8			
9			

3. $K_m = 2 : 4 : 3$

各成分滴加质量见表 4 – 19。

表 4 – 19 $K_m = 2 : 4 : 3$ 时各成分滴加质量

编号	混合表面活性剂/g	GTCC/g	水/g
1			
2			
3			
4			
5			
6			
7			
8			
9			

（二）布洛芬微乳的质量检查

（1）外观性状。

（2）粒径。

（3）离心稳定性。

七、思考题

（1）查阅相关资料，列举 2 种纳米乳的制备方法。

（2）伪三元相图主要包括哪几部分？简述绘制步骤。

（3）滴定过程中，若某次滴水量超过终点而读数不准，是否要立刻倒掉溶液重新做实验？

（4）本实验中不同 K_m 相变曲线有何变化，试分析变化的原因。

参考文献

YOU X H, XING Q, TUO J, et al. Optimizing surfactant content to improve oral bioavailability of ibuprofen in microemulsions: just enough or more than enough? [J]. Int J Pharmaceut, 2014, 471 (1/2): 276 – 84.

实验八　固体脂质纳米粒的制备及评价

一、实验目的

（1）掌握高压均质法和超声辅助微乳法制备固体脂质纳米粒。

（2）熟悉固体脂质纳米粒的质量评价方法。

（3）了解固体脂质纳米粒的其他制备方法。

二、实验原理

1. 固体脂质纳米粒

固体脂质纳米粒（solid lipid nanoparticles，SLN）是近年来迅速发展的一种新型脂质载药系统，是指以固态的天然或合成的类脂如卵磷脂、三酰甘油等为载体，将药物包裹或夹嵌于类脂核中制成粒径在 10～1 000 nm 之间的固态胶粒给药系统。固体脂质纳米粒在室温下通常呈固态，因此具备物理稳定性高、可生物降解、靶向性良好和能大规模生产的优点。SLN 是一种在药剂学研究中常见的制剂亚单元微小实体，如微针或吸入制剂中包载 SLN 实现物理靶向或缓释效果，也可单独制备成混悬剂供口服或注射使用。

2. 常见固体脂质纳米粒制备方法

固体脂质纳米粒骨架材料多为熔点高于室温的脂质材料，有饱和脂肪酸及其甘油酯等，乳化剂可用磷脂和合成乳化剂等。常见的制备方法有高压均质法、微乳法和乳化溶剂挥发法等。本节主要以高压均质法和微乳法为例，介绍固体脂质纳米粒的制备方法。

高压均质法的原理是先将药物与熔融的脂质混合，再将混合物分散至含有表面活性剂的分散介质中，形成初乳。利用高压泵的作用，使初乳通过仅有一个或几个微米的狭缝，在突然减压膨胀和高速冲击碰撞双重作用下，粉碎成乳状微小珠滴。冷却至室温后，即可形成 SLN 分散体系。

微乳法的原理是将脂质载体加热熔融，再加入药物，乳化剂，辅助乳化剂和温水形成外观透明、热力学稳定的 O/W 型微乳，然后在搅拌条件下将微乳分散于冷水中，即可形成 SLN 分散体系。

三、预习思考

（1）查阅相关资料，简述二氟尼柳、布地奈德的理化性质。

（2）查阅相关资料，了解固体脂质纳米粒的常见制备方法。

四、实验材料与仪器

1. 实验试剂与试药
布地奈德、二氟尼柳、三硬脂酸甘油酯、单硬脂酸甘油酯、大豆磷脂、泊洛沙姆188、蒸馏水、无水乙醇。

2. 实验仪器
马尔文粒径分析仪、高压均质机、超声细胞破碎仪、透射电镜、扫描电镜、高效液相色谱仪、烧杯、量筒、容量瓶、天平。

五、实验内容

（一）二氟尼柳固体脂质纳米粒的制备

1. 处方

三硬脂酸甘油酯	300 mg
二氟尼柳	30 mg
泊洛沙姆 188	900 mg
蒸馏水	50 mL

2. 实验步骤
将三硬脂酸甘油酯和二氟尼柳（油相）混合，80 ℃水浴完全熔融；将泊洛沙姆188用50 mL蒸馏水（水相）溶解后，水浴预热至80 ℃。迅速将油相与水相混合后，用高压均质机均质1 min制成初乳。

高压均质机参数设置如下：循环温度为80 ℃，压力设置为1 000 bar。使用前，用80 ℃蒸馏水100 mL预热机器，待温度稳定后，弃去预热用蒸馏水，将初乳倒入高压均质机中，循环10次，收集样品，冷却至室温后即得固体脂质纳米粒分散体系。高压均质机简介详见附录ⅠM。

3. 外观形态
采用透射电镜或扫描电镜观察固体脂质纳米粒的外观形态。

4. 粒径分布
参照粒度和粒度分布测定法（2020版《中国药典》通则0982第三法）测定。取纳米粒混悬液置入马尔文粒径分析仪中，调整稀释倍数，使仪器检测计数率（count rate）为150～300，记录测定的粒径结果。

5. 包封率和载药量的测定
精密吸取5.0 mL制备的纳米粒混悬液，加入10 000 kDa的超滤管中，4 000 r/min

离心 10 min，取滤液，过 0.22 μm 滤膜后，测定其中游离药物含量 A；另精密吸取 5.0 mL 制备的纳米粒，置于 50 mL 容量瓶中，加入无水乙醇使之完全溶解，定容至刻度，测定总药量 B。另取 5.0 mL 纳米粒，干燥后，称量得固体脂质纳米粒总质量记为 W。按照式（4-8-1）和式（4-8-2）分别计算包封率（entrapment efficiency，以 EE 表示）和载药量（drug loading，以 DL 表示）：

$$EE = \frac{B - A}{B} \times 100\% \tag{4-8-1}$$

$$DL = \frac{B - A}{W} \times 100\% \tag{4-8-2}$$

6. 二氟尼柳标准曲线

精密称取二氟尼柳 50 mg 置于 100 mL 量瓶中，用无水乙醇溶解并定容得贮备液。精密量取贮备液适量，分别用无水乙醇稀释至浓度为 1.0 μg/mL、5.0 μg/mL、10.0 μg/mL、15.0 μg/mL、20.0 μg/mL、25.0 μg/mL 和 30.0 μg/mL 的溶液。按高效液相色谱方法测定上述溶液中二氟尼柳的峰面积。以峰面积 A 为纵坐标，浓度 C 为横坐标，进行线性回归，得标准曲线方程。二氟尼柳高效液相色谱条件如下：以十八烷基硅烷键合硅胶为填充剂；以水-甲醇-乙腈-冰乙酸（55∶25∶70∶2）为流动相；检测波长为 254 nm；流速为 1.0 mL/min；进样量为 20.0 μL。

（二）布地奈德固体脂质纳米粒的制备

1. 处方

布地奈德	10 mg
单硬脂酸甘油酯	350 mg
大豆磷脂	120 mg
无水乙醇	5 mL
泊洛沙姆 188	250 mg
蒸馏水	25 mL

2. 实验步骤

将处方量布地奈德、单硬脂酸甘油酯和大豆磷脂，加入 5 mL 无水乙醇，75 ℃ 水浴加热至完全溶解作为油相。将处方量泊洛沙姆 188 溶于 25 mL 水中，75 ℃ 水浴加热至恒温作为水相。将油相在 200 r/min 搅拌条件下缓慢注入水相中，用超声细胞破碎仪对混合后的混悬体系进行超声，功率 100 W，超声 3 s 间隔 1 s，总时间 5 min。超声完毕后，冷却至室温，即得固体脂质纳米粒分散体系。

3. 外观性状、粒径分布、包封率和载药量的测定

外观性状、粒径分布、包封率和载药量的测定参照"五、（一）"中的操作。

4. 布地奈德标准曲线

精密称取布地奈德 50.0 mg 置于 100 mL 量瓶中,用无水乙醇溶解并定容得贮备液。精密量取贮备液适量,分别用无水乙醇稀释至浓度为 1.0 μg/mL、5.0 μg/mL、10.0 μg/mL、15.0 μg/mL、20.0 μg/mL、25.0 μg/mL 和 30.0 μg/mL 的溶液。测定上述溶液在 240 nm 的吸光度。以吸光度 A 为纵坐标,浓度 C 为横坐标,进行线性回归,得标准曲线方程。布地奈德高效液相色谱条件,见吸入粉雾剂章节实验方法。

注意事项

(1) 在使用高压均质机时,要时刻保证高压均质机处于充盈有液体状态,不可进气,否则容易堵塞管道。

(2) 在向高压均质机中倒入混悬溶液前,先使用较高温度蒸馏水对系统预热,以免因为温度过低导致物料析出。

(3) 使用完仪器后要及时用热溶剂清洗,并且在清洗完毕后向仪器中加入约 50 mL 蒸馏水封存。

(4) 使用超声细胞破碎仪时,注意不要让探头触碰到容器底部,以免损伤仪器。

六、实验结果与讨论

(一) 二氟尼柳固体脂质纳米粒的制备

1. 外观形态
采用透射电镜或扫描电镜观察固体脂质纳米粒的外观形态。

2. 粒径分布
记录所制备固体脂质纳米粒的平均粒径及其粒度分布 (表 4-20)。

表 4-20 二氟尼柳固体脂质纳米粒理化性质

粒径	PDI	计数率	zeta 电位/mV

3. 包封率和载药量的测定
绘制二氟尼柳标准曲线,并计算固体脂质纳米粒的包封率和载药量。

(二) 布地奈德固体脂质纳米粒的制备

1. 外观形态
采用透射电镜或扫描电镜观察固体脂质纳米粒的外观形态。

2. 粒径分布
记录所制备固体脂质纳米粒的平均粒径及其粒度分布 (表 4-21)。

表 4 –21 布地奈德固体脂质纳米粒理化性质

粒径	PDI	计数率	zeta 电位/mV

3. 固体脂质纳米粒的包封率和载药量的测定

绘制布地奈德标准曲线,并分别计算固体脂质纳米粒的包封率和载药量。

七、思考题

(1)表面活性剂的用量如何对固体脂质纳米粒的粒径产生影响?

(2)请结合本实验简述固体脂质纳米粒成型过程。

(3)查阅相关资料,简述 3 种常用的固体脂质纳米粒制备方法。

(4)具有哪些理化性质的药物更适合包载在固体脂质纳米粒中?

参考文献

[1] 国家药典委员会. 2020 版中国药典:四部 [M]. 北京:中国医药科技出版社,2020.

[2] 周建平,唐星. 工业药剂学 [M]. 北京:人民卫生出版社,2014:454 – 458.

[3] 雒亚洲,鲁永强,王文磊. 高压均质机的原理及应用 [J]. 中国乳品工业,2007 (10):55 – 58.

第五部分 附 录

附录 I 仪 器

IA 精 密 天 平

【仪器简介】

精密天平是定量分析工作中不可缺少的重要仪器。充分了解仪器性能及熟练掌握其使用方法，是获得可靠分析结果的保证。精密天平的种类很多，有普通精密天平、半自动/全自动加码电光投影阻尼精密天平及电子精密天平等，选择天平应考虑其分度值是否符合称量的准确度要求，其量程是否满足称量要求。称量法主要有 3 种：直接称量法、加重称量法和减重称量法。物品的称量，一般选用称量纸、称量瓶或烧杯等作为容器，当称量的物质具有腐蚀性或挥发性时，称量容器须为密闭容器。

【使用方法】

1. 天平的一般使用流程

（1）将天平置于水平位置，调整天平前面的两个地脚螺栓，直至水平仪内的气泡正好位于圆环的中央。

（2）事先检查电源电压是否匹配（必要时配置稳压器），开机后按仪器要求通电预热至所需时间。

（3）打开天平开关，天平自动进行灵敏度及零点调节。待稳定标志显示后，可进行正式称量。

（4）称量时应从侧门取放物质，读数时应关闭箱门以免空气流动影响天平的稳定性。前门只在检修或清除残留物质时使用。

2. 直接称量法

此法适用于整块物体如整块的金属、器皿或颗粒等的称量，步骤如下：

（1）取一张称量纸叠成铲子（或表面皿），轻轻放在天平托盘上，关上侧门；当显示数字稳定后，按清零键。

（2）将试样置于称量纸或表面皿上，当显示数字稳定后，记录读数。

3. 加重称量法

此法适用于不易吸水、不易氧化或不易与 CO_2 等发生反应的粉末或者小颗粒的称量，步骤如下：

（1）将容器轻轻放在天平托盘上，当显示数字稳定后，按清零键。

（2）加样开始时加入少量试样，一直到接近所需要的药品量时，用拇指和中指及手心拿稳药勺，食指慢慢轻敲药勺柄，让试样慢慢落入器皿中，直到达到要求称取的质量。

4. 减重称量法

此法常用于易挥发或易吸收空气中水或 CO_2 等物质的样品或试剂的称量，也适用于连续称重几份同一试样的质量，试样的质量由 2 次称量之差求得。通过把样品置于密闭的容器（如称量瓶）中称量，能够有效避免由于试样挥发或吸收空气中物质导致试样质量在读数过程中波动，有利于提高称量的准确性。同时，该法能够有效减少试样暴露在空气中的时间，有利于减少试样的变质。步骤如下：

（1）加入适量样品或试剂（约为每份试样量的整数倍）于洁净干燥的称量瓶中，盖好盖子，称出其质量。

（2）取出称量瓶，迅速取出一定量的试样，盖上盖子，再称其质量。前后两次质量之差即为试样的质量。

【注意事项】

（1）天平应放置在牢固平稳水泥台或木台上，在使用天平前，应将水平仪气泡调整至中间位置。室内要求清洁、干燥及较恒定的温度，同时应避免光线直接照射到天平上。

（2）称量结束应及时除去称量瓶（纸），关上侧门，切断电源，并做好使用情况登记。

（3）电子精密天平若长时间不使用，则应定时通电预热，每周 1 次，每次预热 2 h，以确保仪器始终处于良好使用状态。

（4）天平箱内应放置吸潮剂（如硅胶），当吸潮剂吸水变色（蓝色消失），应及时更换。

（5）不易挥发且无腐蚀性的液体称量，常采用烧杯作为容器，可根据实际情况选用加重或减重称量法称量。

（6）具有挥发性、腐蚀性或强酸强碱性的物质应盛于带盖容器（如称量瓶）内称量，以提高称量的准确性，且防止腐蚀天平。

（7）不可过载使用天平。

ⅠB 安瓿熔封机

【仪器简介】

安瓿熔封机采用煤气或石油液化气为燃料，体积小、火焰均匀、拉丝光滑、熔封速度快，工作效率较高，适于注射液试制及学校实验教学用。实验室 RF-J 型安瓿熔封机可对 1～20 mL 规格的安瓿瓶及试管进行熔封。

【组成与构造】

RF-J 型安瓿熔封机集控制箱和熔封台为一体，如图 5-1 所示。前有两个喷火口，后部燃气针型调节阀接口与液化气源相连。

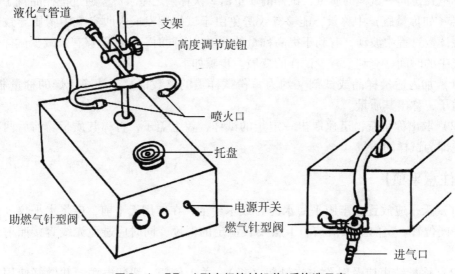

图 5-1 RF-J 型安瓿熔封机前/后构造示意

【使用方法】

（1）将液化气管道通过一个三通阀接到液化气瓶上。

（2）在火焰下方放置一托盘，防止玻璃碎片或液体滴落在仪器上。

（3）连接电源线，开启电源开关。

（4）将液化气管道与气瓶间的三通阀置于"通"的位置。

（5）缓慢开启燃气针型阀，点燃喷火口。

（6）缓慢开启助燃气针型阀，直到两个喷火口发出细长蓝色火焰。

（7）手持安瓿瓶下方，小心将瓶口位于火焰中心，缓慢均匀地转动瓶子使其受热均匀，待烧至软化时，用镊子将安瓿瓶颈上端向上拉断，并将尖头在火焰上稍做灼烧使之熔化圆润，即完成熔封。

（8）工作结束后先关闭助燃气阀门，而后关闭燃气阀门，最后将液化气管道与气瓶间的三通阀置于"闭"的位置。

（9）关闭电源，将电源线拔出。

【注意事项】

（1）液化气瓶必须离熔封机 6 m 以上。

（2）点火时，请勿将身体任何部位暴露于两个喷火口间，以免被火焰烧伤。

（3）点火前必须确认燃气针型阀和助燃气针型阀均处于"关"的位置。然后一边点火一边缓慢开启燃气阀门，点燃后再开启助燃气阀门调节火焰。开启燃气阀门及助燃气阀门时皆应注意速度要缓慢均匀，不可过快，以免火焰爆燃造成事故。

（4）液化气管道与液化气瓶间的三通阀不能有任何泄漏，以免发生事故。

（5）在熔封安瓿时需注意要缓慢转动安瓿瓶，使其受热均匀，待软化后方可用镊子将其向上拉，并在火焰上稍做灼烧，待尖口熔化圆润，以完成熔封。

IC 澄明度检测仪

【仪器简介】

澄明度检测仪适用于灯检法检查各类针剂、大输液和瓶装药液中的可见异物。正确反映制剂澄明度，对于药物生产和科研、保证药品的安全使用，均具有不容忽视的实际指导意义。

【组成与构造】

澄明度检测仪主要由连续传感器、检品盘、检测白板等组成（图 5-2），其光源光照度可在 1 000～4 000 lx 范围内调节，无色供试品溶液检查时的光照度应为 1 000～1 500 lx，正面不反光的黑色面作为检查无色或白色异物的背景，侧面和底面的白色面作为检查有色异物的背景。

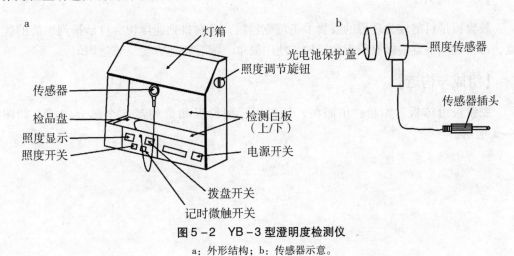

图 5-2 YB-3 型澄明度检测仪
a：外形结构；b：传感器示意。

【使用方法】

（1）启动澄明度检测仪的电源开关。

（2）启动照度开关，此时照度显示为数字："00"表示照度为 0×100 lx。

（3）将传感器放置在测定检品位置测定照度，同时调节仪器上部旋钮，调至所需照度条件，照度调好后，拔下插头，关闭照度开关。

（4）根据所测样品要求，用拨盘开关设定所需检测的时间。

（5）如需控制检测时间，在检测样品的同时，按动计时微触开关，指示灯每 6 s 闪烁 1 次，且起始和终止有报警声响。

（6）测试完毕后，关闭仪器总电源，拔下电源插头。

【注意事项】

（1）仪器使用前一定要检查电源插座的地线是否可靠接地，检品盘内若有药水应及时清除，以防流入电源箱内造成其他事故。

（2）打开电源后，若灯管不亮首先检查保险管和电源，调节仪器灯管旋钮时禁止旋转 360°，最大只能旋转 180°，以防止灯管接触不良。

（3）检查人员远距离和近距离视力测验，均应为 4.9 或 4.9 以上（矫正后视力为5.0 或 5.0 以上）；应无色盲。

（4）检查时，检查人员应调整位置，使供试品位于眼部的明视距离处（指供试品至人眼的距离，通常为 25 cm）。

（5）除另有规定外，置供试品于遮光板边缘处，在黑色背景下，用目检视，再在白色背景下检视 1 次。

ID　胶 囊 板

【仪器简介】

胶囊板是目前较为理想的胶囊手工填充器械，具有排列速度快、自动排列率高的优点，可避免用手直接接触胶囊和药粉，使用简单、灌装快速方便、装量均匀。

【组成与构造】

胶囊板由体板、帽板、中间板、压粉板、刮粉板和排列盘 6 个部分组成，如图5-3 所示。

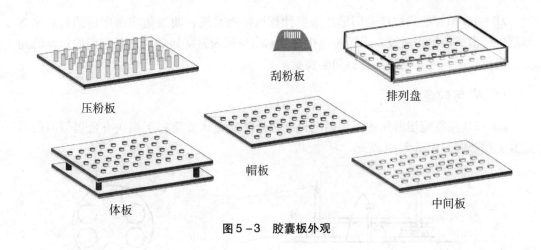

图 5-3　胶囊板外观

【使用方法】

（1）装胶囊体。体板平整放好，排列盘边框朝上置于体板上，再将空胶囊体放入排列盘边框内，拿起体板和排列盘左右摆动，胶囊体会一一掉入体板。体板装满后，将多余胶囊体通过排列盘边框豁口倒出，取走排列盘。将装好胶囊体的体板置于一边待用。

（2）装胶囊帽。将体板换成帽板，胶囊体换成胶囊帽，执行第一步操作。

（3）胶囊体装粉。根据每次填充的胶囊粒数和每粒胶囊的装量，使用天平称取胶囊内容物，置于装好胶囊体的体板上，用刮粉板在体板上来回刮至装满，最后刮去体板上多余药粉。

（4）胶囊体与胶囊帽锁扣。将中间板无缺口的一面对准放到帽板上，使帽板中胶囊帽口高出帽板面的部分进入中间板的孔中，然后两板一起翻转180°，对准放到体板上来回轻轻推压几下，使胶囊帽口与体口稍微结合，然后将整套板翻转使帽板向下、体板向上，再用力压紧。待都压到底后，翻转胶囊板，拿掉帽板，取出中间板，将锁合好的胶囊从中间板上倒出。

【注意事项】

（1）清洁胶囊板后，应再用纯化水冲洗，置桌面自然晾干，严禁烘箱加热干燥。

（2）填充胶囊时，应保持实验台面干净，保持胶囊板干燥，胶囊壳不得沾水。

ⅠE　崩　解　仪

【仪器简介】

崩解仪主要用于检查片剂、胶囊剂、丸剂等口服固体制剂在规定条件下的崩解情况。

ZB－1D 型智能崩解仪采用单片微型计算机控制系统，通过集成温度传感器对水浴温度进行恒温控制，通过 2 个同步电机带动两组吊篮做升降运动，并对它们的运动时间分别进行控制，可分别独立进行崩解实验。

【组成与构造】

ZB－1D 型智能崩解仪主要包括主机、能升降的金属支架和下端镶有金属筛网的吊篮等主要部件，如图 5－4 所示。

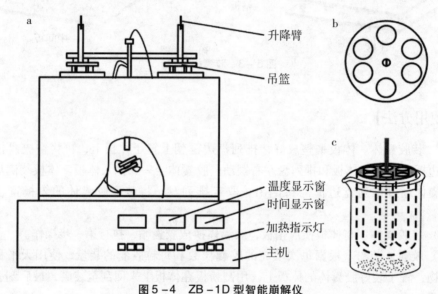

图 5－4　ZB－1D 型智能崩解仪

a：崩解仪外形结构示意；b：吊篮俯视；c：吊篮侧视。

【使用方法】

（1）开机。确认水浴槽已注水到规定高度后打开电源，温度显示窗显示当前的温度修正值，约 5 s 后，恢复显示实测水温值；左右时间显示窗显示"0：00"；气泵开始工作，水浴槽内砂块冒出气泡，仪器处于待机状态。

（2）温度预置与控温。预置温度确认无误后，按"启/停"键，仪器进入加热控温状态，当水浴温度达到预置温度并稳定于恒温状态后，方可开始试验。

（3）时间预置与控制。该仪器具有左、右两组吊篮，可分别独立进行崩解实验，与之对应的左右两个时间窗可分别显示出各自的实验实时或预置时间。通过时间控制"＋""－""启/停"键可进行时间的预置和试验的各种操作。

（4）准备溶液。按升降键，使吊臂停在最高位置，以便装取烧杯和吊篮，将各烧杯分别注入所需的实验溶液，然后装入水浴槽杯孔中；再将各个吊篮分别放入烧杯内，并悬挂在支臂的吊钩上。

（5）崩解实验。将供试品放入吊篮的各个玻璃管内，必要时放入挡板（注意排出挡板下面的气泡，以免其浮出液面）；然后按时间控制的"启/停"键，吊篮开始升降运动。观察各吊篮玻璃管中供试品的崩解状况。预置时间到后，吊篮自动停在最高位置。

（6）结束实验。关闭电源，从水浴槽中取出烧杯与吊篮，处理溶液，清洗干净，收置备用。

【注意事项】

（1）水浴槽中无水时，严禁启动加热，否则会损坏加热器。

（2）主机箱后方、水浴槽上方有连接塑料管的尼龙单向阀，防止水槽中的水虹吸倒流，不可接反（接反亦无气泡产生）。

ⅠF 透皮扩散试验仪

【仪器简介】

透皮扩散试验仪是适用于经皮给药制剂体外经皮渗透实验的实验设备，通过将离体的皮肤（或人工膜）夹在扩散池中，角质层面向给药池，将药物置于给药池中，于给定的时间间隔测定皮肤另一侧接收池内的药物浓度，分析药物经皮渗透的动力学。此外，可用于预测药物经皮吸收的速度，研究介质、处方组成和经皮吸收促进剂等对药物经皮渗透速度的影响。

【组成与构造】

透皮扩散试验仪主要包括扩散池及恒温水浴等部件，RYJ-6B 透皮扩散试验仪的结构及外形如图 5-5 所示。

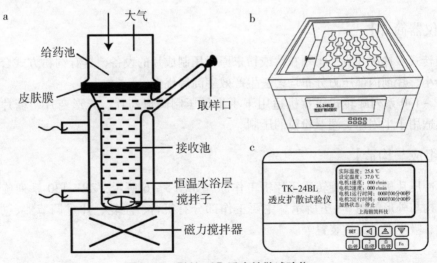

图 5-5 RYJ-6B 透皮扩散试验仪

a：扩散池；b：透皮扩散仪外观；c：控制面板。

【使用方法】

（1）将仪器内部装满干净的蒸馏水，并安装好温度探头，确认水循环系统正常，正确安装挡板。

（2）打开电源开关，根据实验设定温度，同时打开加热开关。

（3）将配制好的扩散液加入扩散池中。

（4）将扩散池组装好，给药池和接收池中间加入扩散膜，接收池中加入1个转子，然后用弹簧夹夹紧，并将其逐一置于扩散池的内架上。

（5）根据实验设计转速并开启。

（6）开始进行体外经皮渗透实验，从底部扩散池取出样品溶液，然后再补加入同等温度、体积的扩散介质溶液。

（7）实验结束清洗各个部件及设备，归于原处存放。

【注意事项】

（1）安装温度探头需通过挡板小孔并浸没于水中，水循环系统应浸没于水中，且吸附于仪器内壁，严禁水箱内无水时开机。

（2）样品溶液取样以及补样需要保证接收池与扩散膜之间没有气泡，以免导致透皮面积不准确，可以采用注射器配软管取样，同时用长针针管进行补液。

（3）仪器不用时应将水放尽，将给药池与接收池清洗干净，同时将搅拌子存于储存袋中，置于通风处。

IG　旋转式多冲压片机

【仪器简介】

旋转式多冲压片机是将颗粒状或粉末原料压制成片的设备，具有饲粉方式合理、片重差异小、片剂内部压力分布均匀、生产效率高等优点。

ZP-130系列旋转式压片机适用于小批量压制圆形药片、异形药片、糖片、钙片等，不适用于半固体、潮湿粉粒的压制。

【组成与构造】

单冲压片机与多冲旋转式压片机工作原理如图5-6所示，ZP-130系列旋转式压片机结构与外形如图5-7所示。主要工作部分有机台、压轮、片重调节器、加料斗、饲粉器、吸尘器、保护装置等。

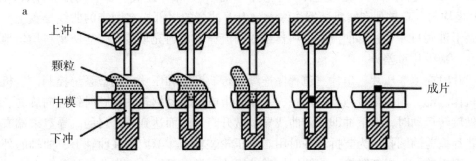

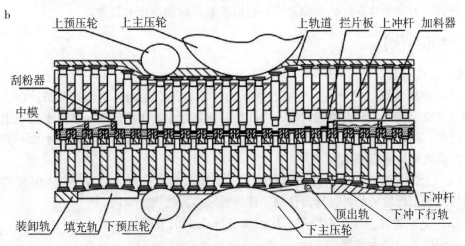

图 5-6　单冲压片机与多冲旋转式压片机的工作原理示意

a：单冲压片机原理图；b：旋转式压片机原理图。

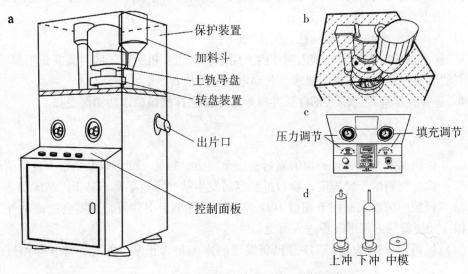

图 5-7　ZP-130 旋转式压片机结构示意

a：旋转式压片机外观；b：压片机上部俯视放大图；c：控制面板；d：上冲、下冲、中模。

ZP－130 旋转式压片机的上冲、中模、下冲三个部分连成一体，周围 5 副、7 副、9 副冲模均匀分布排列在转盘装置边缘上，上下冲杆的尾部嵌在固定的曲线导盘上。采用由腰形锥底料斗和月形回流式加料器组成的流栅式加料充填装置，能使物料均匀地充满模孔，减少片重差异。

压片时充填、压片、出片三道程序连续进行。充填和压片由调节系统控制，电机安装在机体底部，用三角带拖动减速箱，工作时由电机传动蜗轮轴做顺时针方向旋转。当转盘做旋转运动时，上下冲即随着曲线导盘做升降运动而达到压片目的。导盘末端有一被圆垫片掩盖的圆孔，为装拆下冲时用。下压轮装在主体槽内套在曲轴上，曲轴的外端装有 1 副蜗轮，与蜗杆联接，旋转蜗杆带动蜗轮而做微量转动。当曲轴的偏心向上，压轮上升，压力增加片薄，减少则片厚，借以控制片剂的厚度和硬度。

【使用方法】

1）冲模安装：

（1）中膜装置。打开顶面封板，拆下加料器架，料斗加料器，打开防护门，用手转动减速箱手轮，使转台慢慢转动。当孔位转到靠近上冲上行轨时，拆下上行轨上的嵌块。同时，用打模棒穿过上冲孔轻轻将中模打入中模腔，中模平面与转台平面平齐为合格，然后将螺钉紧固依次装入。

（2）上冲装置。通过上行轨的嵌块处，冲杆尾部涂机械油插入，插入时使冲杆尾部的槽对准上行轨的凸处，转台移动，逐件插入后再把嵌块紧固。

（3）下冲装置。打开中间门，从主体的圆孔中取下圆垫，装法与上冲相同，下冲安装完毕后必须装上圆垫片。

（4）冲模全套装毕后，用手继续转动手轮，使转盘旋转 1～2 转，观察上下冲进入中模孔和在曲线导轨上的运行，必须灵活无碰撞和剐蹭现象，开动电机空车运动 2～3 min，平稳正常即可使用。

2）检查颗粒或粉末的流动性，倒入加料斗。

3）初次试压应先将物料倒入料斗内，用手转动压片机手轮，同时调节充填和压力，使片剂的质量和硬度达到成品要求，开动电机进行压片。

4）压片完毕应及时清洗部件，冲模等零部件涂抹机械油以防潮湿受损。

【注意事项】

（1）使用前须重复检查冲模的质量，应无缺边、裂缝、变形以及紧松不合等情况。

（2）检查物料的干燥程度，物料过湿容易发生粘冲，过干则不易于固结成型。

（3）颗粒中的粉末最好不超过 10%，颗粒不宜小于 100 目，否则会造成粘冲、原料耗损，并使机件内部因飞粉进入而受损。

（4）仪器运行过程中随时注意机器发出的声响是否正常，如有异常立即停机进行检查。

（5）加料斗堵塞：若颗粒细小、黏性或湿度较大、流动不畅，会使加入膜孔颗粒减少，影响片重。若遇片重突然减小时，应立即停机检查。

（6）片重差异较大：颗粒过湿，细粉过多，颗粒粗细不均，以及颗粒中润滑剂不足，均能引起片重差异较大，这时应从提高颗粒质量着手。

（7）片剂硬度和重量差异合格的前提下，压片过程中应每隔 10～20 min 检查片剂质量。

（8）压片完毕，应用粉剂刷清理机器各部位的残留细粉。如停用时间较长，必须将冲模全部拆下，并将机器全部揩擦清洁。

IH　高效包衣机

【仪器简介】

高效包衣机是对药片、药丸进行糖衣、水相薄膜、有机薄膜包衣的专用设备。整个工艺操作过程在密闭状态下进行，无粉尘飞扬和包衣液飞溅，是一种优质高效、可靠、洁净、节能、操作方便的新型包衣设备。

【组成与构造】

高效包衣机主要由风路系统（进风管、加热箱、过滤器、进风斗、锅体、排风斗、风机）、喷雾系统和控制系统三部分组成，如图5-8所示。

电机带动锅体做圆周运动。片芯在锅体导流板及防滑条带动下，不停地做循环翻滚运动。雾化喷枪连续向片床层喷洒包衣材料。同时，在可控的负压状态下，热风不断经过片床层并由底部排出，使片芯表面包衣材料快速、均匀干燥，从而形成一层坚固、致密、平整、光滑的外膜。

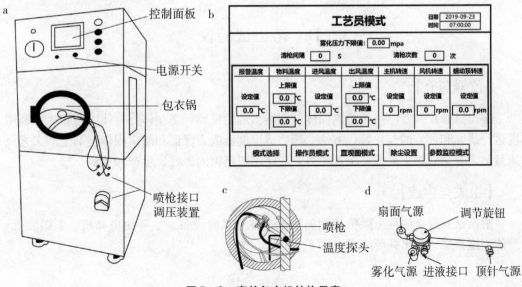

图5-8　高效包衣机结构示意
a：包衣机外观；b：控制面板；c：包衣锅内部；d：喷枪。

【使用方法】

（1）风路系统。安装顺序为进风斗、锅体、排风斗，安装时，轻转部件对准卡槽，顶紧，拧紧卡箍（3个），注意排风斗胶皮在锅体外部。

（2）喷枪系统。安装喷枪与水平面呈45°，与片床面平行，卡在最高处，温度探头触及片床。

（3）控制面板。进入"工艺员模式"进行参数设置。

（4）开启主机、风机、加热装置，待物料温度上升至设定区间，开启顶针气源、雾化气源、蠕动泵，使喷枪喷出雾滴。

（5）喷入包衣液直至片面色泽均匀一致，增重至处方量，关闭蠕动泵、雾化气源、顶针气源，再加热2 min后关闭加热开关，待报警温度降至40 ℃以下后关闭风机与主机，关闭包衣机电源。

（6）拆卸并清洗锅体、进风斗、排风斗和喷枪系统。

【注意事项】

（1）包衣液现配现用，配制时防止产生大量气泡，使用过程中保持持续轻微搅拌状态，以防止产生沉淀。

（2）要求素片较硬、耐磨，包衣前要用风筒吹去素片上的细粉，使片面光洁。

（3）包衣操作中，应注意控制物料温度和进风温度，温度过高则干燥太快导致成膜不均匀，温度太低则干燥太慢造成粘连。

（4）喷液速度及包衣锅转速应适宜，速度过快易出现成膜不均匀、磕片现象。

（5）包衣中途可使用长柄药勺取样观察，尽量不打开密封门。

（6）包衣结束后应及时清洗喷枪系统，防止残余包衣液凝结堵塞系统。

II　溶出试验仪

【仪器简介】

溶出试验仪是专门用于检测固体制剂溶出度的仪器，是在体外对体内药物生物利用度进行研究和评价的有效替代方法。药物溶出度已成为保证和衡量固体制剂生产工艺及质量是否合理和稳定的重要检查项目，广泛用于药物的研究、生产和检测。

【组成与构造】

溶出试验仪是一种由微机控制的机电一体化试验设备，主要由电动机、恒温装置、篮体、搅拌桨、溶出杯等组成（图5-9）。

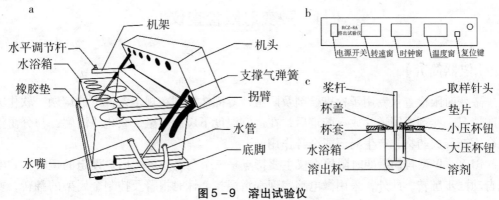

图 5-9 溶出试验仪

a：溶出仪外观；b：控制面板；c：溶出杯。

【使用方法】

（1）安装溶出杯。将溶出杯分别放入杯架板各杯孔内，将转轴倒置，插入各轴孔中，向下伸出。利用中心盖检查溶出杯是否与轴同心。若不同心，可调节水槽位置使溶出杯与轴同心。

（2）接通电源：按开机座右侧电源开关，3 个显示窗（转速、时间和温度）均亮。

（3）取出 1 个溶出杯，在恒温水槽中加去离子水至红色标线，按温度显示屏下按钮设置恒温温度后，启动水浴升温。

（4）将转轴由下向上插入各轴孔中，将定位球依次放入 6 个溶出杯，缓慢压下转轴，使转轴底部接触定位球中央。

（5）将离合器端口内有拨齿一端朝下分别从转轴上端套入，下移使拨齿落入轴套的凹槽中，小心顺时针拧紧离合器，固定住已经用定位球调节好的 6 个转轴的高度。

（6）注入已经超声处理的溶出介质，盖好保温盖。

（7）长按溶出仪"设置"键至计时或限时模式，设定相应时间和转速，待温度到达设置温度并保持稳定，投入样品，启动转轴旋转，仪器自动开始计时。

（8）到达取样时间点时，用注射器连接杯盖的针头取样（长针头适用于桨法测定，短针头适用于小杯法测定），针头应从取样孔插入并下降至最低处，保证取样位置在桨叶顶端至液面的中点，距溶出杯内壁不小于 10 mm 处。每次取样后须立即补充相同体积的空白溶出介质。

（9）溶出结束后关闭电源，取下杯盖，掀起设备上层，清洁桨叶及溶出杯。如果较长时间不用，须放空恒温水槽中的水。

【注意事项】

（1）切勿在缺水时接通电源。

（2）盖好保温盖，不宜过早预热溶出介质，以免蒸发。

（3）勿使用有机溶剂清洗仪器外壳。

IJ 融变时限检查仪

【仪器简介】

融变时限检查仪专用于检查栓剂及阴道片等固体制剂在规定条件下的熔融、软化或溶解情况。栓剂或阴道片放入腔道后，在适宜温度下应能熔融、软化或溶解，与分泌液混合逐渐释放药物，产生局部或全身作用。

RBY - IV型自动融变时限检查仪主要特点是三个金属架可按用户设定的运转方式实现自动同步翻转。此外，采用微电脑实现水浴温控、计时报警及控制金属架的翻转，操作简单，性能优良，符合国家药典的规定。

【组成与构造】

RBY - IV融变时限检查仪由主机箱和水浴箱两部分组成，如图5-10所示。仪器主机箱的前面板设有数字式时间显示窗和温度显示窗，另有加热指示灯、电源开关及6个功能键。时间显示窗中央的"双点"在计时中每秒闪烁1次，右边显示秒值，左边显示分值。温度显示窗在初始设置时显示P1、P2或P3三种时限方式（选择其一）以及预定温度，在运行后显示实际水温，所显示的温度值精确到0.1 ℃。

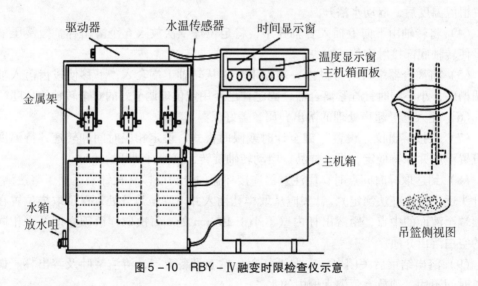

驱动器　水温传感器　时间显示窗　温度显示窗　主机箱面板　金属架　主机箱　水箱放水咀　吊篮侧视图

图5-10　RBY - IV融变时限检查仪示意

【使用方法】

（1）水箱注水。不放烧杯时，将水加至红色水线处，放入套好胶圈的烧杯后（加不少于4 L的水），时间显示为00：00，温度显示为实际水温。

（2）时限选择。P1：运行30 min，套筒每隔10 min自动翻转1次，适用于油脂性基质的栓剂测试；P2：运行60 min，套筒每隔10 min自动翻转1次，适用于水溶性基质的栓剂；P3：运转30 min，套筒不翻转，适用于阴道片测试。

（3）温度预定。利用温度设定键预定温度。根据药典对药样的测试温度要求，仪器已预定水浴工作温度为 37 ℃。

（4）控温。温度预定好后按温控键，此时加热器运行，显示实际水温。

（5）辅助。在加热期间，为使烧杯中水温均匀，套筒可每分钟翻转 1 次，起到搅拌作用，通过辅助键来实现；到预定温度后，再按 1 次辅助键可取消翻转。

（6）栓剂测试。供试品在室温下放置 1 h 后方可使用。双手托起桥板，取出金属架。将 3 粒供试品分别放入 3 个金属架的下层圆盘上，装入各自的套筒内后，将桥板放回水箱上，按测试键进行测试。

【注意事项】

（1）通电后显示不正常，即时间显示不是 00：00 或温度显示不是实际水温，应关闭电源再接通。

（2）水箱未注水时严禁开机，否则水泵易损坏。

（3）水循环系统工作不正常时，严禁按温控键加热，否则电热管易烧毁，导致主机损坏。

（4）水浴温度升到预定值时，杯中水温会有滞后，加热时间可适当延长再次测试。

（5）长期不使用时，应将水浴箱中的水放干净。

（6）桥板的升降应轻托轻放，避免冲撞、跌落等情况。

IK　热熔挤出机

【仪器简介】

热熔挤出技术（hot-melt extrusion）是指通过加热和剪切作用，将药物和辅料熔融混合，使药物高度分散在固体载体材料中的技术，是制备固体分散体的新技术。

热熔挤出机主要由计算机控制系统、加料系统、挤压传动系统、加热冷却系统和下游辅助加工系统构成。按照原理不同，挤出机可分为柱塞式和螺杆式。柱塞式挤出机的温度均匀性和混合能力较差，已逐步被螺杆式挤出机取代。螺杆式挤出机根据螺杆的不同，可分为单螺杆、双螺杆和多螺杆挤出机。

【使用方法】

热熔挤出技术操作简单。操作前将机筒预热至设定温度，药物和辅料预混。挤出过程分四步（图 5 - 11）：①通过加料系统添加物料；②在螺杆的作用下，熔融、混合；③传送；④所得产品从机头口模挤出或进入下游装置。

与传统的制剂技术相比，热熔挤出技术具有以下优点：①制备过程无须使用溶剂或水，绿色环保，避免湿度敏感药物的降解；②药物均匀分散在载体中，含量均一；③工艺简单，可连续生产，适合产业化；④方便赋形。但热熔挤出过程使用的温度较高，所以药物和辅料需要具有较好的热稳定性，故不适用于热敏性药物和蛋白多肽类药物。

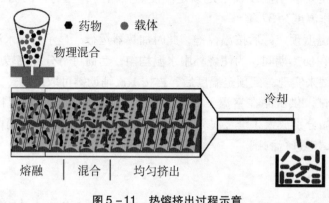

图 5 - 11　热熔挤出过程示意

IL　超细微粒制备系统

【仪器简介】

超细微粒制备系统（ultrafine particle preparation system，UPPS）是一种前景广阔的新型微球制备技术。相较于传统的乳化法、复乳法，无须大量的乳化剂，药物包封率高；相较于喷雾干燥法，条件温和，有利于维持活性成分的稳定。后处理无须水洗、离心、冷冻干燥等多重间歇步骤，工艺简单，可实现自动化连续生产。

【组成与构造】

超细微粒制备系统主要由供液系统、旋碟系统、气流系统、温控系统、液氮供应器、控制系统和样品收集器等组成。

【使用方法】

（1）将药物和载体制成溶液、乳状液或悬浮液。

（2）液体的微滴化与分散。混合液体定量喷射到高速旋转的碟片后，在离心力作用下由中央向外周运动，受旋碟刻纹影响铺展为一层薄的液膜。液膜在碟片边缘被剪切雾化为微滴，抛射进入设备腔内气流。

（3）微滴的固化。微滴随气流运动，在气－液界面张力的作用下，保持表面自由能最低的球体形状。溶剂逐渐挥发，微滴固化成微球。或经过特定的载气或载液处理后，形成微球。

（4）微球的收集与处理。微球固化后，由于重力逐渐沉积于样品收集装置。

【注意事项】

制备微球时，需要选择合适的供液速度和旋碟转速。

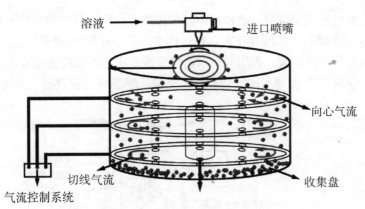

图 5 - 12　UPPS 工作原理示意

IM　高压均质机

【仪器简介】

高压均质机是一种常见的物料均质仪器。其均质过程短，物料分散均匀度高，应用范围广，在制药领域可用于脂质体、纳米乳剂、纳米混悬剂等的制备，是目前最有效的纳米颗粒制备仪器之一。

【组成与构造】

高压均质机主要由高压均质腔和增压机构组成。以高压往复泵为动力传递和物料输送机构，将液态物料或以液体为载体的固体颗粒输送至高压均质腔部分。物料在通过高压均质腔的过程中，在高压下产生的高速剪切、高频震荡、对流撞击、空穴现象和湍流涡旋等机械力作用和相应的热效应下超微细化。

Niro Soavi NS1001L 2K 型高压均质机由泵体（压缩头、柱塞泵、吸放球阀）、压力表、均质阀、进料口、物料杯、出料口构成（图 5 - 13），可在高达 1 500 bar[①] 的压力下处理各种黏度的物料，特别适用于实验室处理小批量样品。

【操作方法】

（1）预处理液体样品。

（2）检查进料口及物料杯中有无异物，进样口中加入热溶剂预热高压均质机。打开电源开关及压力表开关，以零压力冲洗管路。缓慢转动二级阀，检查是否能到达 100 bar，后缓慢旋松二级阀，使压力为 50 bar。缓慢转动一级阀，检查是否能到达 1 000 bar，观察有无异常。

（3）预热完成后，排放进样室中用于预热仪器的热溶剂至仅剩约 20 mL 时，迅速加入预热的样品，以避免仪器运行过程中进入空气。同时调节均质压力，使其稳定在所

---

① 　1 bar = 0.1 MPa。

需压力。待柱塞中的残留溶剂从出料口中基本排出后，开始收集均质后的样品。

（4）按规定步骤完成实验操作后，在进样室内样品仅剩约 20 mL 时，加入约 50 mL 预热洗涤溶剂循环洗涤 5 次，再用蒸馏水清洗管路 3 次，注意应完全弃掉洗涤溶液。然后加入 20%～30% 乙醇循环 1 次，使管路中充满乙醇溶剂封存仪器，关闭电源。

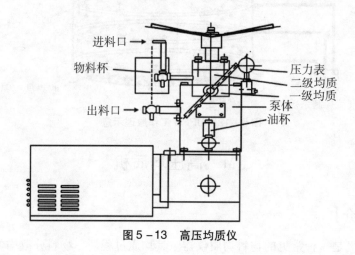

图 5-13　高压均质仪

【注意事项】

（1）高压均质机不得直接进样固体样品，物料在均质前应先过滤，以免损坏仪器。

（2）高压均质机使用过程中，保证进料口内有液体，以防泵入空气（样品中空气含量应该小于 2%），否则影响均质效果并损坏仪器。

（3）若仪器发生堵塞，需对仪器进行洗涤后再进行实验。

（4）调压过程中，应缓慢旋转均质阀，以免损坏密封圈，导致样品泄露。

（5）使用过程中禁止关闭温控系统，且温度不宜超过 85 ℃。

（6）仪器使用完毕应及时按照流程清洗仪器。

附录Ⅱ　辅料（包衣材料）

ⅡA　全配方薄膜包衣系统欧巴代®

欧巴代®（Opadry®）是卡乐康®（Colorcon®）公司全配方薄膜包衣材料系统的商品名。Opadry®薄膜包衣配方提供水性和有机溶剂两种包衣工艺。水性薄膜包衣是

Colorcon® 的主要特色，其将成膜材料、增塑剂、着色剂等混制成一个干粉系统，该干粉系统于包衣前加水配制成包衣液使用。Opadry®薄膜包衣液配制如下。

1. 实验材料与仪器

Opadry®薄膜包衣系统、水（去离子水或蒸馏水）、可调速搅拌机、螺旋桨式搅拌桨（搅拌桨的直径应等于配液容器直径的 1/3～1/2）、配液容器（体积应比所要配制的液体总量大 15%～25%）。

2. 包衣液配制与使用

（1）在配液容器中加入所需量的溶剂，水做分散介质最高可配制固含量为 15%～20% 的包衣液。液体高度应当等于或稍大于容器的直径。一般推荐包衣增重为 2%～3%。

（2）将搅拌桨置于容器的中央，并尽量靠近容器的底部。搅拌溶剂使其形成一个旋涡，但要避免卷入空气。

（3）将 Opadry®粉末均匀地加入旋涡中，同时避免有粉末飘浮在液体表面。必要时，可以提高转速保持适当的旋涡。

（4）待所有的 Opadry®粉末全部加入后，降低搅拌速度致使旋涡几乎消失，继续搅拌 45 min。

（5）配制好的包衣液可以通过蠕动泵，直接从配液容器中泵出至喷枪使用。

（6）整个包衣过程中，包衣液始终维持轻微搅拌状态。

ⅡB　包衣材料尤特奇®

尤特奇（Eudragit®）是合成药用辅料的商品名，它包括甲基丙烯酸共聚物和甲基丙烯酸酯共聚物，在中国被称为丙烯酸树脂类药用辅料。Eudragit®应用广泛，可作为药物制剂的胃溶包衣、肠溶包衣、缓控释包衣、保护隔离包衣、缓释骨架材料和经皮给药制剂的骨架胶粘材料。

（一）Eudragit®产品种类

各种 Eudragit®均由几种单体聚合而成，常用产品见表 5-1。

表 5-1　Eudragit®产品汇总

商品名	化学组成	形态	注册名称	用途
E100	甲基丙烯酸丁酯、甲基丙烯酸二甲胺基乙酯和甲基丙烯酸甲酯（1：2：1）共聚物	颗粒	甲基丙烯酸氨烷基酯共聚物 E 型	防护型包衣
E PO		粉末	—	
L 100-55	甲基丙烯酸和丙烯酸乙酯（1：1）共聚物	粉末	甲基丙烯酸共聚物 C 型	十二指肠释药
L 30D-55		30% 水分散体	甲基丙烯酸 - 丙烯酸乙酯共聚物水分散体	

续表 5 – 1

商品名	化学组成	形态	注册名称	用途
L 100	甲基丙烯酸和甲基丙烯酸甲酯（1∶1）共聚物	粉末	甲基丙烯酸共聚物 A 型	空肠释药
S 100	甲基丙烯酸和甲基丙烯酸甲酯（1∶2）共聚物	粉末	甲基丙烯酸共聚物 B 型	结肠释药
FS 30D	甲基丙烯酸、丙烯酸甲酯和甲基丙烯酸甲酯（1∶1∶1）共聚物	30% 水分散体	—	
RL 100	丙烯酸乙酯、甲基丙烯酸甲酯和甲基丙烯酸氯化三甲胺基乙酯（1∶2∶0.2）共聚物	颗粒	季胺基甲基丙烯酸酯共聚物 A 型	缓释配方
RL PO		粉末	—	
RL 30D		30% 水分散体	—	
RS 100	丙烯酸乙酯、甲基丙烯酸甲酯和甲基丙烯酸氯化三甲胺基乙酯（1∶2∶0.1）共聚物	颗粒	季胺基甲基丙烯酸酯共聚物 B 型	
RS PO		粉末	—	
RS 30D		30% 水分散体	—	
NE 30D	丙烯酸乙酯和甲基丙烯酸甲酯（2∶1）共聚物	30% 水分散体	丙烯酸乙酯 – 甲基丙烯酸甲酯共聚物水分散体	

注：灰色背景为常用 Eudragit®。

（二）Eudragit®水分散体

Eudragit®水分散体是一种粒度为 0.01 ~ 0.10 μm 的聚合物乳胶粒在水中的分散体，聚合物的质量分数为 30%，黏度低，易于喷雾包衣操作。成膜过程中，乳胶粒形成堆积层，随水分蒸发，表面张力增大，使胶粒紧密聚集，在最低成膜温度以上环境中形成薄膜。这种膜的抗水渗透性优于用有机溶剂包衣液形成的膜，并且水散体包衣有利于安全生产和环境保护。

以滑石粉为抗黏剂配制的 Eudragit®水分散体包衣液，常用柠檬酸三乙酯作为增塑剂，辅料配比见表 5 – 2。

表 5 – 2　Eudragit®水分散体包衣液辅料配比

Eudragit®	L30D-55	FS 30D	NE 30D	RL／RS 30D
滑石粉（Talc）（相对于聚合物的质量）	50%	50%	50% ~ 100%	50%
柠檬酸三乙酯（TEC）（相对于聚合物的质量）	10%	5%	—	20%
包衣液固含量	20% ~ 25%			

Eudragit®水分散体包衣液配制步骤：

（1）Eudragit®水分散体包衣液的配制如图5-14所示，将滑石粉和柠檬酸三乙酯加入水中，用高剪切均质机匀化10 min。必要时加入少量（0.5%）的消泡剂（如二甲基硅油）。

（2）将滑石粉混悬液缓慢倒入Eudragit®水分散体中，同时用搅拌机中速搅拌不少于30 min。

（3）混悬液过40目筛，保持轻微搅拌状态，备用。

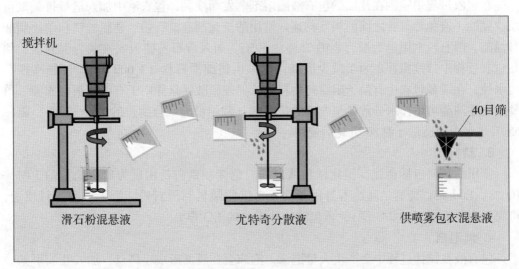

图5-14 Eudragit®水分散体包衣液的配制

（三）Eudragit®的溶解特性

常见Eudragit®的溶解特性见表5-3。

表5-3 Eudragit®的水溶性

商品名	水溶解性
L/S	含有羧基，在水中很容易与碱生成盐而溶解； Eudragit® L 100 在 pH 大于 6 的溶液中溶解；Eudragit® S 100 在 pH 大于 7 的溶液中溶解
E100	在近中性（pH 为 5～7）环境中不溶解，在 pH 小于 5 的介质中很快溶解； 具有叔胺基，强亲水性，在 pH 为 5 以上的介质中有较大的溶胀性，可崩解
RL/RS	在水中不溶，但能溶胀，在包衣中形成孔道； 在生理 pH 范围内（pH 为 1～8），盐溶液的浓度影响包衣材料溶胀

（四）Eudragit®常用添加剂

1. 增塑剂

增剂塑可提高薄膜的柔韧性，有助于喷雾液滴在片面铺展和相互结合，有利于完整薄膜的形成。增塑剂对水分散体更是不可缺少，它能降低聚合物的成膜温度，使水分散体中的聚合物乳胶粒在包衣操作温度下或在包衣后热处理过程中融合成致密的薄膜。常用的增塑剂有柠檬酸三乙酯、柠檬酸三丁酯和癸二酸二丁酯等。柠檬酸三乙酯性质稳定也最为常用。增塑剂的合适用量为聚合物的 10%～20%。过量增塑剂会增加薄膜的黏性，应该避免。用 Eudragit® L 和 Eudragit® S 水分散体包衣时，由于其玻璃化温度较高，为了将成膜温度降至室温，应加入 40%～50% 增塑剂。

2. 抗黏剂

在包衣过程中喷洒在片面的包衣液随溶剂蒸发而变黏，包衣液中加入适量抗黏剂可减少黏性，避免片与片之间的相互粘连。常用的抗黏剂有滑石粉、硬脂酸镁和单硬脂酸甘油酯。滑石粉常用量为聚合物的 25%～50%。加入滑石粉使包衣液成为混悬液，须在包衣过程中持续搅拌。为了减少沉降，宜采用超细滑石粉（1 000 目）。硬脂酸镁有疏水性，在缓释包衣中有助于阻滞药物释放，但硬脂酸镁只能用于有机溶剂包衣液。单硬脂酸甘油酯可用作水分散体包衣液的抗黏剂，常用量为聚合物量的 2%～10%，需在65 ℃热水中加适量吐温 80 乳化后使用。

3. 颜料

常用的颜料包括色淀、氧化铁和钛白粉。色淀和钛白粉用量为聚合物量的 10%～100%，Eudragit® 能容纳高达本身用量 2～3 倍的颜料和滑石粉。为了节省颜料用量，可先包无色内层（约 2/3 厚），再包着色外层（约 1/3 厚）。

4. 消泡剂

包衣液在搅拌过程中会产生大量泡沫，泡沫会在膜面形成小斑点，加入几滴甲基硅油可消除或减少泡沫。消泡有利于包衣的致密性。消泡剂加入量为聚合物量的0.1%～0.5%。

附录Ⅲ 评 价 方 法

ⅢA 革兰氏染色

【原理】

结晶紫初染和碘液媒染会在细胞壁内形成不溶于水的紫色复合物。对革兰氏阳性菌染色时，由于其细胞壁较厚、肽聚糖网层次较多且交联致密，乙醇脱色处理时肽聚糖网孔因失水而缩小，导致结晶紫–碘复合物被截留在细胞壁内，使细菌呈紫色；相比之下，革兰氏阴性菌具有细胞壁薄、外膜层类脂含量高、肽聚糖网层薄且交联度差等特点，遇乙醇脱色时，以类脂为主的外膜迅速溶解、薄而松散的肽聚糖网无法阻挡结晶紫–碘复合物的溶出，此时呈现无色。再经蕃红等红色染料复染，革兰氏阴性菌显红色。

【实验步骤】

革兰氏染色法一般包括初染、媒染、脱色、复染 4 个步骤，具体操作方法如下：

（1）涂片，火焰固定。

（2）草酸铵结晶紫染色，1 min 后水洗。

（3）加碘液覆盖涂面染色，1 min 后水洗。

（4）滴加 95% 酒精，轻轻摇动进行脱色，30 s 后水洗。

（5）蕃红染液染色，1 min 后水洗。

（6）干燥，镜检。

注意：每次水洗后应使用滤纸吸去多余水分。

【结果观察】

革兰氏阴性菌显红色，革兰氏阳性菌显紫色。本实验容易出现假阳性和假阴性的结果，影响因素如下：

（1）涂片过厚或者结晶紫染色过度，都会导致脱色不完全，导致假阳性结果的出现。判断应以均匀分散开的细菌染色结果为准。

（2）细菌固定过度导致的细胞壁通透性增大，或者细菌培养时间过长导致的部分细胞死亡或自溶，最终都会引起假阴性结果。

【注意事项】

（1）标本涂片不宜过厚。若涂片较厚，应适当延长脱色时间。

（2）固定玻片时，火焰温度不宜过高。

（3）水洗动作轻柔，沿载玻片对角线方向或反面冲洗，避免把菌体冲掉。

ⅢB 显微镜标尺的计算与标定

在显微镜下，通常使用测微尺来测量物体大小。由于显微镜之间放大倍数存在差异，故在测量物体之前必须标定目镜的测微尺，其结构及测量方法如图 5 – 15 所示。

1. 目镜测微尺的标定

目镜测微尺放在目镜的横格上，物镜测微尺放于载物台上。通过显微镜观察，保持两把测微尺平行，左端刻度对齐重合后，寻找两者再次重合的刻度位置，分别记录格数。根据物镜测微尺的长度（已知）以及目镜测微尺和物镜测微尺的换算关系计算目镜测微尺每格所代表的实际长度。

2. 物体大小的测定

取走物镜测微尺，将待测样品置于载物台上。在显微镜下观察，缓慢移动样品。用目镜测微尺测量物体的直径或长度，根据所占格数可换算出实际尺寸。

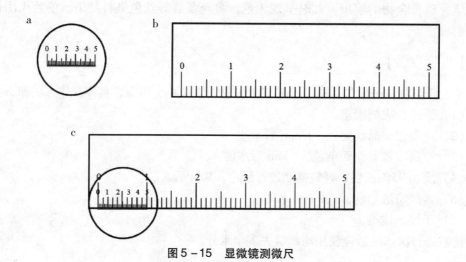

图 5 – 15　显微镜测微尺

a：目镜测微尺；b：物镜测微尺；c：测量示意。

ⅢC　吸入制剂递送剂量均一性和微细粒子空气动力学特性测试

1. 递送剂量均一性（吸入气雾剂和吸入粉雾剂）测试

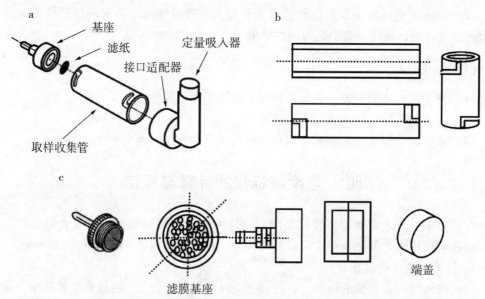

图 5 – 16　递送剂量均一性（吸入气雾剂和吸入粉雾剂）测定装置

a：装置组装结构简图；b：取样收集管；c：测试装置。

测定装置如图 5 – 16 所示，包括一个带有不锈钢筛网、用以放置滤纸的基座，1 个配有两个密封端盖的取样收集管和 1 个吸嘴适配器，以确保取样收集管与吸嘴间的密封性。该装置能定量收集吸入气雾剂的递送剂量。

采用合适的适配器确保气雾剂吸嘴端口与样品收集管口或 2.5 mm 的缩肩平齐。在基座内放入直径为 25 mm 的圆形滤纸，固定于取样收集管的一端。基座端口连接真空泵、流量计。连接测定装置和待测气雾剂，调节真空泵使其能够以 28.3 L/min 流速从整套装置抽气，包括滤纸和待测气雾剂。空气应持续性从装置抽出，避免活性物质损失进入空气。组装后装置各部件之间的连接应具有气密性，从取样收集管中抽出的所有空气经过待测吸入剂。

2. 吸入制剂微细粒子空气动力学特性测试

雾滴（粒）分布和微细粒子剂量是评价吸入制剂质量的重要参数。吸入制剂的雾滴（粒）大小，在生产过程中可以采用合适的显微镜法或光阻、光散射及光衍射法进行测定；但产品的雾滴（粒）分布，则应采用雾滴（粒）的空气动力学直径分布来表示。2020 版《中国药典》规定了 3 种装置（双级撞击器、安德森圆盘撞击器、新一代撞击器）来评价粒子的空气动力学特性。这里简单介绍新一代粒子撞击器（next generation impactor，NGI）。

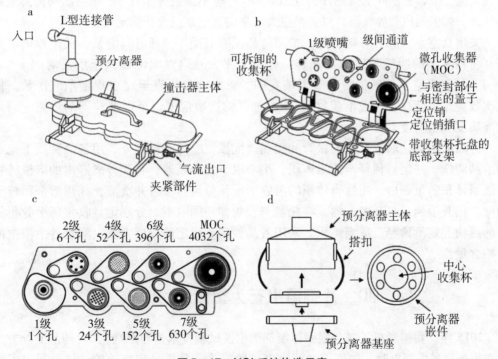

图 5 - 17 NGI 系统构造示意

a：NGI（安装了预分离器）；b：NGI 组件；c：NGI 的喷嘴配置；d：预分离器配置。

新一代粒子撞击器结构如图 5 - 17 所示，是具有 7 级和 1 个微孔收集器（micro-orifice contactor，MOC）的级联撞击器。将 L 型连接管与装置入口相连，选用合适的吸嘴适配器以保证吸入剂和 L 型连接管之间的气密性。对于粉雾剂，一般应在 L 型连接管和撞击器间加预分离器。若经实验验证不引起级间药物损失增加（大于 5%）或颗粒二次夹带，则可省略预分离器。若样品含有大量不能被末端 MOC 收集的颗粒，可以用滤纸装置替代 MOC 或置于 MOC 下端（可使用玻璃纤维滤纸）。为确保能够有效地收集颗粒，可将甘油、硅油或其他合适液体溶于挥发性溶剂中，在每级收集杯表面进行涂层（除非实验证明不需要）。

对于吸入粉雾剂的测定，将收集杯置于托盘内，将托盘安装于底部支架上，保证各收集杯对应底部支架相应位置。合上盖子，扳下手柄，将仪器密封。将预分离器嵌件组装至预分离器基座内，将预分离器基座安装到撞击器入口，在预分离器嵌件中心收集杯内加入各品种项下规定的溶剂 15 mL，安装预分离器主体，扣紧。

在撞击器入口端或预分离器入口端插入 L 型连接管，在 L 型连接管的另一端安装合适的吸嘴适配器。粉雾剂吸嘴插入后，驱动器的吸嘴端应在 L 型连接管的水平轴线上，吸嘴的端口应与 L 型连接管口平齐。与吸嘴适配器相连后，粉雾剂的放置方向应与实际使用方向一致。将装置与流量系统相连。除另有规定外，在 L 型连接管进口气体流速为 Q_{out}（Q_{out} 的测定见吸入粉雾剂的制备与评价章节）的条件下测试。开启真空泵，将流量计连接到 L 型连接管处，调节流量控制阀使通过系统的稳定流量达到 Q_{out}（±5%）。在测试流量下，控制阀前后的压力比（P_3/P_2）应小于或等于 0.5，即控制阀内形成临界气流。如未形成临界气流，可更换更大功率的真空泵或重新测定流量。

关闭真空泵。除另有规定外，按照药品说明书操作。开启真空泵，关闭双向电磁阀，将粉雾剂的吸嘴与适配器相连，保持水平，开启双向电磁阀至所需时间 t（±5%），通过真空泵抽气将粉末吸至装置中。重复此过程直至完成规定抽气次数。抽气次数应尽可能少，一般不超过 10 次，抽气的次数应能保证微细粒子剂量测定结果的准确度和精密度。

拆除撞击器，取下 L 型连接管和吸嘴适配器，除另有规定外，用各品种项下规定的溶剂清洗，并定量稀释至适当体积。小心取下预分离器，将预分离器内的溶液转移至适当体积的量瓶内，用适当体积的溶剂清洗预分离器，合并洗液，并用溶剂稀释至刻度。松开手柄，打开撞击器，将托盘与收集杯一同取下，分别定量收集每个收集杯内的药物并定量稀释至适当体积。采用各品种项下规定的分析方法，测定各溶液中的药物含量。

ⅢD　片剂溶出行为相似性的比较

2015 年，我国颁布了《口服固体制剂溶出度试验技术指导原则》，对药品的处方工艺在批准后发生变更时，如何通过溶出度试验确认药品质量和疗效的一致性提出了建议。固体制剂口服给药后，药物的吸收取决于药物从制剂中的溶出或释放、药物在生理条件下的溶解以及在胃肠道的渗透。由于药物的溶出和溶解对吸收具有重要影响，因此体外溶出度试验有可能预测其体内行为。该文件对于普通口服固体制剂的体外溶出评价及体内溶出相关性等问题提出了具体的指导意见，对国内药物开发和仿制药一致性评价具有重要意义。其中，关于溶出曲线相似性的比较，不仅对新药及仿制药的开发具有重要意义，同时对药剂学的研究也有重要参考意义。

1. 非模型依赖的相似因子法

采用相似因子（f_2）来比较溶出曲线是一种简单的非模型依赖方法。通过式（5-3-1）计算 f_2：

$$f_2 = 50 \lg \left\{ \left[1 + \frac{1}{n} \sum_{t=1}^{n} (R_t - T_t)^2 \right]^{-0.5} \times 100 \right\} \qquad (5-3-1)$$

式中，n 为取样时间点个数，R_t 为参比样品（或变更前样品）在 t 时刻的溶出度值，T_t 为试验批次（变更后样品）在 t 时刻的溶出度值。

相似因子的测定过程，一般分为两步。首先，分别取受试（变更后）和参比样品（变更前）各 12 片（粒），测定其溶出曲线。然后，取两条曲线上各时间点的平均溶出度值，根据上述公式计算相似因子（f_2）。f_2 值越接近 100，则认为两条曲线的相似性越高。一般情况下，f_2 值高于 50，可认为两条曲线具有相似性，受试（变更后）与参比产品（变更前）具有等效性。这种非模型依赖方法最适合于三四个或更多取样点的溶出曲线比较，但采用本方法时应满足下列条件：

（1）应在完全相同的条件下对受试和参比样品的溶出曲线进行测定。2 条曲线的取样点应相同。

（2）应采用变更前生产的最近一批产品作为参比样品。

（3）药物溶出量超过 85% 的取样点不超过 1 个。

（4）第一个取样时间点的溶出量相对标准偏差不得超过 20%，其余取样时间点的溶出量相对标准偏差不得超过 10%。

（5）当受试制剂和参比制剂在 15 min 内的溶出量 ≥85% 时，可以认为两者溶出行为相似，无须进行 f_2 的比较。

2. 非模型依赖多变量置信区间法

对于批内溶出量相对标准偏差大于 15% 的药品，可能更适于采用非模型依赖多变量置信区间方法进行溶出曲线比较。建议按照下列步骤进行：

（1）测定参比样品溶出量的批间差异，然后以此为依据确定多变量统计矩（multivariate statistical distance，MSD）的相似性限度。

（2）确定受试和参比样品平均溶出量的多变量统计矩。

（3）确定受试和参比样品实测溶出量多变量统计矩的 90% 置信区间。

（4）如果受试样品的置信区间上限小于或等于参比样品的相似性限度，可认为 2 个批次的样品具有相似性。

3. 释放模型拟合

在仿制药一致性评价过程中，除了比较溶出曲线相似性外，还可以对释放模型进行拟合，比较自研制剂和参比制剂的释放机制，从而预估生物等效性（bioequivalency，BE）风险。

常见的溶出拟合数学模型见表 5-4。

表 5 −4 常见溶出拟合数学模型

模型名称	模型方程	模型参数定义
零级释放模型	$Q = k_0 \cdot t$	Q 为累积释放百分率；t 为时间
一级释放模型	$Q = 100 \times [\, 1 - e^{-kt}\,]$	Q 为累积释放百分率；t 为时间
Higuchi 模型（曲折孔道扩散）	$Q = k_H \cdot t^{0.5}$	Q 为累积释放百分率；t 为时间；k_H 为溶解常数
Korsmeyer-Peppas 模型（多重释放机制）	$Q = k_{KP} \cdot t^n$	Q 为累积释放百分率；t 为时间；k_{KP} 为释放常数，n 为与形状相关的释放参数，$n \leqslant 0.45$，以扩散为主；$0.45 < n < 0.89$，存在扩散和溶蚀两种行为，$n \geqslant 0.89$，则以溶蚀为主，尤其适用于释放机制不明确的制剂